CANCER ETIOLOGY, DIAGNOSIS AND TREATMENTS

# MANTLE CELL LYMPHOMA

# CLINICAL CHARACTERISTICS, PREVALENCE AND TREATMENT OPTIONS

# Cancer Etiology, Diagnosis and Treatments

Additional books in this series can be found on Nova's website under the Series tab.

Additional e-books in this series can be found on Nova's website under the e-book tab.

CANCER ETIOLOGY, DIAGNOSIS AND TREATMENTS

# MANTLE CELL LYMPHOMA

# CLINICAL CHARACTERISTICS, PREVALENCE AND TREATMENT OPTIONS

CHARLES L. SCHMIDT
EDITOR

*New York*

**Library of Congress Cataloging-in-Publication Data**

ISBN: 978-1-63482-363-0
Library of Congress Control Number: 2015933899

*Published by Nova Science Publishers, Inc. † New York*

# Contents

# Preface

This book discusses the clinical characteristics of mantle cell lymphoma, as well as its prevalence and examines several treatment options available.

Chapter 1 – Mantle cell lymphoma (MCL) is a morphologically, phenotypically, and genetically well-defined mature B-cell neoplasm with an aggressive clinical course. MCL was first recognized as "centrocytic lymphoma" by the Kiel classification due to resemblance of the lymphoma cells to the germinal center centrocytes. Later, "lymphocytic lymphoma of intermediate differentiation, mantle zone lymphoma" as defined by the localization of lymphoma cells in the mantle zones of secondary lymphoid follicles was found to have morphologic and phenotypic overlap with the "centrocytic lymphoma". These early immunophenotypical studies also excluded the derivation of the "centrocytic lymphoma" from germinal center B-cells. The finding of strong association of t(11;14)(q13;q32)/translocation of CCND1 (also known as BCL1 or PRAD1) with these lymphomas confirmed that these lymphomas represented a distinct lymphoma entity, and allowed recognition of the different morphologic variants. The term "mantle cell lymphoma" was first proposed by the International Lymphoma Study Group (ILSG) in 1992. The diagnostic criteria proposed by ILSG were later incorporated into the Revised European-American Lymphoma Classification and then to the World Health Organization (WHO) Classification of Tumours of Haematopoietic and Lymphoid Tissues. In the 2008 WHO classification, MCL is defined as a "B-cell neoplasm generally composed of monomorphic small to medium-sized lymphoid cells with irregular nuclear contours and a CCND1 translocation. Neoplastic transformed cells (centroblasts), paraimmunoblasts and proliferation centres are absent", and the diagnosis of MCL is based on the characteristic morphology, immunophenotypic features, presence of cyclin D1 protein overexpression and/or t(11;14)(q13;q32)/IGH-CCND1 translocation. However, more recent gene expression profiling studies revealed the existence of a small subset of MCLs with negative cyclin D1/CCND1 translocation. The wide clinical spectrum of MCL ranging from indolent to highly aggressive variants was also well recognized.

Chapter 2 – Mantle cell lymphoma (MCL) is a subtype of Non-Hodgkin's Lymphoma (NHL) with varying clinical presentations, ranging from indolent disease to highly aggressive clinical course. The MCL cells exhibit a characteristic translocation t(11;14) which juxtaposes immunoglobulin heavy chain gene with gene for cyclin D1 leading to overexpression of cyclin D1 which can be identified by immunohistochemistry and is useful as a diagnostic marker. Advancement in understanding of the biology and pathogenesis of MCL has led to discovery of multiple other genetic alterations impacting the cell cycle deregulation and development of sub clonal populations with certain genetic mutations (p53, ATM, NOTCH2) leading to disease progression and refractoriness to treatment. Mantle cell lymphoma international prognostic index (MIPI) and biologic MIPI (bMIPI) are prognostic indices to categorize indolent vs aggressive disease. Currently an intensive cytarabine containing upfront induction regimen followed with or without autologous transplant is recommended for younger and fit patients. Older or frail patients are thought to benefit more from less intensive rituximab containing regimens followed by rituximab maintenance. A small subset of patients with indolent disease can be observed. Most patients unfortunately relapse. Targeted molecular therapies (bortezomib, lenalidomide, ibrutinib, idelalsib etc.) have shown significant response rates in relapsed and refractory disease and are being evaluated further.

Chapter 3 – Mantle cell lymphoma (MCL) is a type of non-Hodgkin lymphoma characterized by an indolent histologic picture but an aggressive clinical course. The cytogenetic marker of MCL is chromosomal translocation t(11;14) (q13; q32), with expression of cyclin D1. As MCL remains incurable, modification of its treatment represents an important challenge. The introduction of rituximab, more intensive chemotherapy and the increasing use of autologous stem cell transplant (ASCT) in first remission has results in some improvement in the survival of MCL patients. Recently, several targeted agents have shown promising activity in MCL, of which lenalidomide, proteasome inhibitors or m-TOR inhibitor were found to be efficient in relapsed and refractory disease, even when used as a single agents. Moreover, B-cell receptor pathway inhibitors such as ibrutinib and idelalisib have also shown high activity, since abnormalities in this pathway are believed to be crucial in MCL pathogenesis. Similarly, histone deacetylase (HDAC) or cyclin-dependent kinase inhibitors have shown some promise in early phase trials. In this review the authors present the state of the art for emerging targeted therapies for MCL.

Chapter 4 – The complex network of the malignant B cell with the tumor microenvironment and the constitutive activation of the B-cell receptor pathway promote survival and proliferation of malignant B cells. The downstream targets of the BCR pathway and the microenvironment are the other mediators of cell growth in B cell lymphoma. Recently, small molecule inhibitors that inhibit BCR associated pathways have shown encouraging activity in B cell lymphoma. The B cell receptor pathway therefore, has become an attractive prime target in several incurable lymphomas such as chronic lymphocytic leukemia and mantle cell lymphoma. The growing body of knowledge on the efficacy of these agents and yet the lack of a comprehensive understanding of the potential targets and off target actions is intriguing.

In this chapter, the authors will review the safety, mechanism of action, efficacy and future directions of the targeted therapies in the management of mantle cell lymphoma.

Chapter 5 – Mantle cell lymphoma (MCL) is an uncommon non-Hodgkin (NHL) lymphoma subtype with distinct features in terms of its clinical presentation and prognosis which are usually characterized by diffuse extranodal disease, including spleen and bone marrow involvement as well as an intermediate to high MCL international prognostic score. Elucidation of MCL underlying molecular aberrations not only resulted in the emergence of a key role for cyclin D1 and intracellular protein turnover regulation but has also introduced a rational of targeted therapeutic approaches, of which proteasome inhibitors have become an essential part. Bortezomib is the first proteasome inhibitor which was established as part of FDA-approved therapy for relapsed/refractory MCL in 2006. Since then much progress has been noted with accumulating preclinical and early clinical evidence suggesting additive or/and synergistic activity of bortezomib and newer proteasome inhibitors with cytotoxic and targeted agents, including but not limited to rituximab, histone deacetylase inhibitors, mTOR inhibitors and cyclin-dependent kinase inhibitors. A growing number of combination studies are currently under progress in MCL patients with the aim of better understanding and framing the use of proteasome inhibitors in the continuum of treatment approaches for the management of MCL.

In: Mantle Cell Lymphoma
Editor: Charles L. Schmidt

ISBN: 978-1-63482-363-0


Chapter 1

# Diagnosis, Prognosis and Genetic Features of Mantle Cell Lymphoma

***Haipeng Shao****

Department of Hematopathology and Laboratory Medicine
H. Lee Moffitt Cancer Center and Research Institute, Tampa, FL, US

Mantle cell lymphoma (MCL) is a morphologically, phenotypically, and genetically well-defined mature B-cell neoplasm with an aggressive clinical course. MCL was first recognized as "centrocytic lymphoma" by the Kiel classification due to resemblance of the lymphoma cells to the germinal center centrocytes. [1] Later, "lymphocytic lymphoma of intermediate differentiation, mantle zone lymphoma" as defined by the localization of lymphoma cells in the mantle zones of secondary lymphoid follicles was found to have morphologic and phenotypic overlap with the "centrocytic lymphoma". [2-6] These early immunophenotypical studies also excluded the derivation of the "centrocytic lymphoma" from germinal center B-cells. The finding of strong association of t(11;14)(q13;q32)/translocation of CCND1 (also known as BCL1 or PRAD1) with these lymphomas confirmed that these lymphomas represented a distinct lymphoma entity, and allowed recognition of the different morphologic variants. [7-14] The term "mantle cell lymphoma" was

* Tel: 813-745-2672; E-mail: Haipeng.Shao@moffitt.org.

first proposed by the International Lymphoma Study Group (ILSG) in 1992. [15] The diagnostic criteria proposed by ILSG were later incorporated into the Revised European-American Lymphoma Classification and then to the World Health Organization (WHO) Classification of Tumours of Haematopoietic and Lymphoid Tissues. [16, 17] In the 2008 WHO classification, MCL is defined as a "B-cell neoplasm generally composed of monomorphic small to medium-sized lymphoid cells with irregular nuclear contours and a CCND1 translocation. Neoplastic transformed cells (centroblasts), paraimmunoblasts and proliferation centres are absent", [17] and the diagnosis of MCL is based on the characteristic morphology, immunophenotypic features, presence of cyclin D1 protein overexpression and/or t(11;14)(q13;q32)/IGH-CCND1 translocation. However, more recent gene expression profiling studies revealed the existence of a small subset of MCLs with negative cyclin D1/CCND1 translocation. [18] The wide clinical spectrum of MCL ranging from indolent to highly aggressive variants was also well recognized. [19-23]

## Epidemiology and Clinical Features

MCL accounts for approximately 3-10% of non-Hodgkin lymphomas with an incidence of 0.55 per 100,000 in the United States. [24, 25] It usually occurs in elderly individuals with a median age of close to 70 years at the time of diagnosis, and shows a male predominance with male to female ratio of 2.3-2.5:1. [26] Most patients with MCL present with systemic disease with generalized lymphadenopathy, splenomegaly, and bone marrow involvement (Ann Arbor stage III-IV disease). Peripheral blood is frequently involved by MCL, and 92% patients show peripheral blood involvement by flow cytometry. [27] Extranodal sites are frequently involved, including the gastrointestinal tract, which is involved in >90% patients with MCL, even in endoscopically unremarkable mucosa. [28] A distinctive form of primary MCL of the GI tract is termed multiple lymphomatous polyposis, with the appearance of many sessile or pedunculated polyps on the small and large intestinal mucosa. [29] Patients with multiple lymphomatous polyposis often present with abdominal pain, diarrhea and weight loss. [30] Although multiple lymphomatous polyposis represents MCL in most cases, it may also represent follicular lymphoma and MALT lymphoma. [30-35]

MCL is aggressive and incurable with median survival of 3-5 years. [36] Recently, two clinically indolent variants of MCL have been recognized. The first is a leukemic MCL with lymphocytosis in the peripheral blood, low-level interstitial bone marrow involvement, splenomegaly, and slow or absent clinical progression. [22] The second is the so called "in situ" MCL, which is often an incidental finding and associated with very indolent clinical course. [20] On the other end of the spectrum, the blastoid and pleomorphic variants of MCL are associated with aggressive clinical course. A rare but highly aggressive variant of MCL has been recognized and is characterized by concurrent MYC gene rearrangement or amplification. [21, 23]

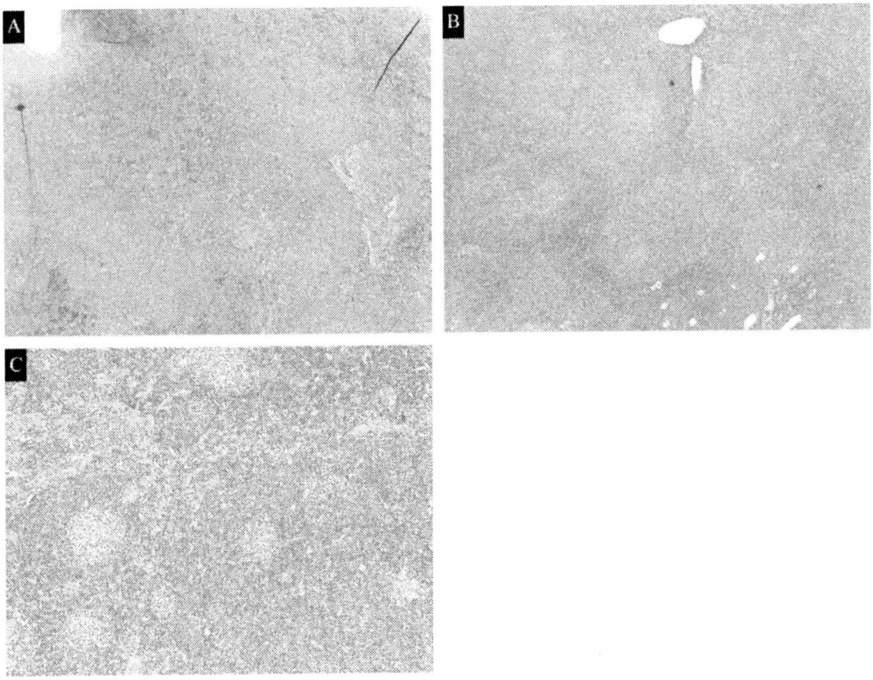


Figure 1. Mantle cell lymphoma growth pattern. (A), diffuse (B), nodular (C) mantle zone.

# Morphologic and Immunophenotypic Features

Classic MCL shows lymphoid infiltrate composed of a monotonous population of small to medium-sized lymphoid cells with irregular nuclei, mature chromatin, inconspicuous nucleoli and scant cytoplasm, resembling centrocytes. [15, 17, 37] Prolymphocytes, paraimmunoblasts, centroblasts and immunoblasts are absent. In the lymph node, there are three main growth patterns: diffuse, vaguely nodular and mantle zone (Figure 1). [4, 15, 38, 39] Many cases show a combination of the diffuse and vaguely nodular patterns. In the diffuse pattern, the lymph node architecture is effaced by sheets of small to medium-sized atypical lymphoid cells often associated with scattered epithelioid histiocytes (Figure 2A and 2B). Hyalinized blood vessels also may be present. In the nodular pattern, the lymph node shows effaced architectures by large numbers of vague lymphoid nodules composed uniformly of MCL cells. The lymphoid nodules resemble primary lymphoid follicles and do not contain germinal centers or separate distinct mantle zones. In both the diffuse and vaguely nodular patterns, proliferation centers characteristic of chronic lymphocytic leukemia/small lymphocytic lymphoma are absent. In the mantle zone pattern, the lymph node architecture is usually not completely effaced by atypical lymphoid follicles with variably expanded mantle zones surrounding residual germinal centers. Of the three main patterns, diffuse pattern is most frequently seen and mantle zone pattern is least common. [37] MCL typically does not show plasmacytic differentiation, although rare cases of MCL with nodular and mantle-zone growth pattern and t(11;14) positive clonal plasma cells have been reported. [40]

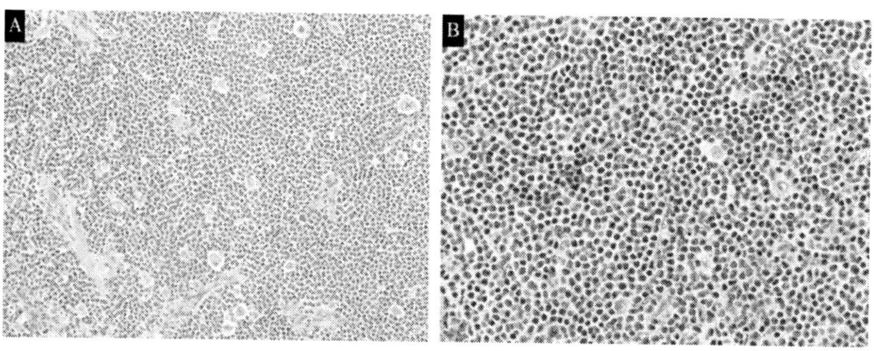


Figure 2. Classic mantle cell lymphoma. (A), sheets of small lymphoid cells with scattered epithelioid histiocytes and hyalinized vessel (left lower side of the picture) (B), cells of classic MCL are small with mildly irregular nuclei, coarse chromatin and scant cytoplasm.

There are four morphologic variants of MCL recognized by the 2008 WHO classification: blastoid, pleomorphic, small cell and marginal zone-like. [17] The blastoid and pleomorphic variants are aggressive variants and must be recognized and documented in the pathology report due to the association with poor prognosis. The small cell and marginal zone-like variant may cause diagnostic challenge with incomplete study. The blastoid MCL is characterized by medium-sized lymphoid cells with finely dispersed chromatin, cytologically resembling lymphoblasts (Figure 3), and frequently associated with high mitotic figures (usually >20-30/10 high power field). The pleomorphic MCL cells are medium-sized to large with oval to pleomorphic nuclei, vesicular chromatin and often prominent nucleoli, resembling diffuse large B-cell lymphoma. The small cell MCL demonstrates small lymphoma cells with round nuclei, dense chromatin and scant cytoplasm, cytologically resembling cells of chronic lymphocytic leukemia/small lymphocytic lymphoma. [41] The small cell MCL variant has been reported to represent an indolent disease with bone marrow involvement, splenomegaly and lower proliferation rate. [42] The marginal zone-like MCL is rare and characterized by foci of MCL cells with abundant pale cytoplasm, resembling marginal zone-cells or monocytoid B-cells.

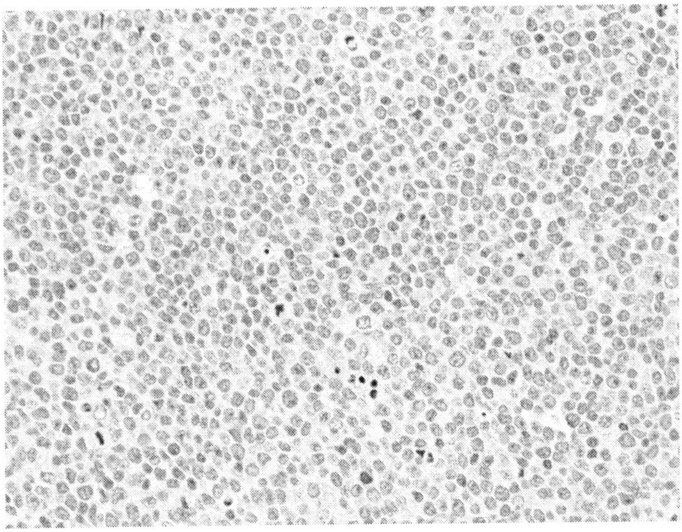

Figure 3. Blastoid mantle cell lymphoma. The cells of blastoid MCL have fine chromatin and associated with frequent mitotic figures.

Unlike other low grade small B-cell lymphomas, such as follicular lymphoma, marginal zone lymphoma or chronic lymphocytic leukemia/small lymphocytic lymphoma, MCL does not undergo transformation to diffuse large B-cell lymphoma. Approximately 20-30% cases of classic MCL undergo blastoid transformation during the course of the disease or at relapse, and most cases of blastoid and pleomorphic MCL occur *de novo*. [43, 44]

In the spleen involved by MCL, the spleen is markedly increased in size and the cut sections show a miliary pattern with numerous tiny white nodules or larger fleshy white nodules. Large mass lesions are typically absent. Microscopically, spleen shows predominantly white pulp involvement and variably red pulp infiltrate by MCL cells (Figure 4). The white pulp is expanded by nodules of small to medium-sized MCL cells. Mantle zone pattern may be present in some cases with residual germinal centers. Occasional cases may show a marginal zone pattern, raising the differential diagnosis with splenic marginal zone lymphoma. [45, 46] The splenic lymph nodes are almost always involved in patients with splenic MCL.

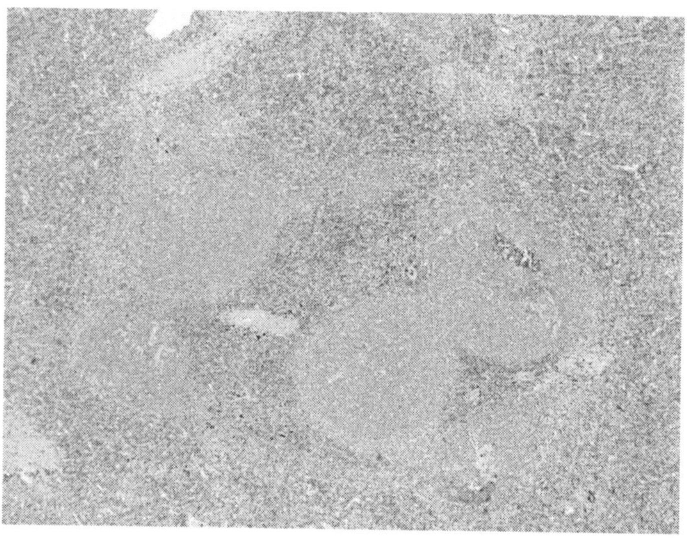

Figure 4. Mantle cell lymphoma in spleen. The spleen shows predominantly white pulp involvement by MCL with a nodular pattern.

Multiple lymphomatous polyposis of the GI track takes the form of many fleshy white polyps on the mucosa surface of small and large intestines. MCL may present grossly as discrete masses, ulcers, and mucosal thickenings. [47] Microscopically, the polyps consist of vague nodules of MCL cells in the mucosa. Residual germinal centers may be seen in some of these neoplastic nodules, giving rise to the mantle zone growth pattern. The MCL cells may invade the superficial submucosal areas. Lymphoepithelial lesions and marginal zone differentiation is absent. In patients with nodal MCL, most (approximately 90%) also show GI involvement by MCL, usually at microscopic level even in the grossly unremarkable mucosa. [28, 48] This microscopic involvement is usually patchy and has little impact on clinical management of the patients. [48]

On peripheral blood smears, the MCL cells are typically small to medium-sized with irregular to cleaved nuclei, mature chromatin and inconspicuous nucleoli (Figure 5). In leukemic blastoid MCL, the peripheral blood shows many medium-sized atypical lymphoid cells with blast-like fine chromatin, resembling acute leukemia. [49] In the very aggressive MCL with MYC gene rearrangement or amplification, the lymphoma cells are large with round to irregular nuclei, blast-like chromatin, prominent nucleoli and moderate amounts of basophilic cytoplasm, some with cytoplasmic vacuoles, which cytologically resemble leukemic diffuse large B-cell lymphoma. [21] A small subset of leukemic MCL shows >55% prolymphocyte-like lymphoid cells in the peripheral blood. These cases were previously diagnosed as B-cell prolymphocytic leukemia, but are now classified as MCL based on the presence of t(11;14)(q13;q32). [50-54]

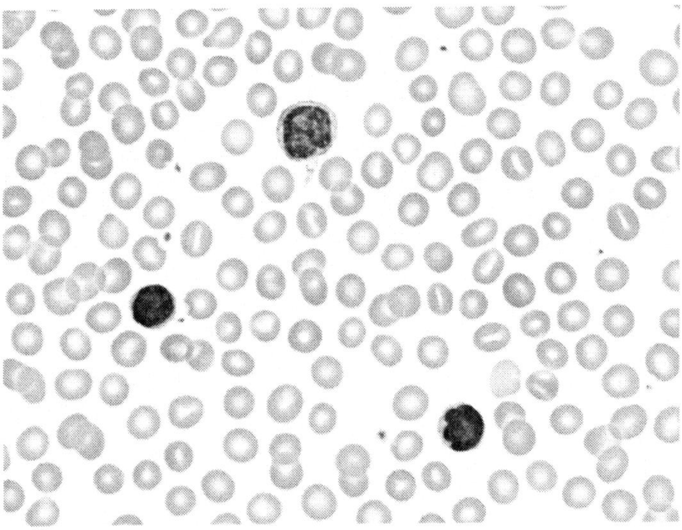

Figure 5. Mantle cell lymphoma in peripheral blood. The cells of MCL are small to medium in size with mildly irregular nuclei and mature chromatin.

Bone marrow is frequently involved by MCL. The infiltration patterns in the bone marrow by MCL are nodular (most common, Figure 6), interstitial, paratrabecular and diffuse (least common). [55, 56] The lymphoma cells show similar cytological features as that of nodal MCL. The blastoid MCL tends to show interstitial or diffuse pattern in the marrow and cytologically resembles acute leukemia. [57]

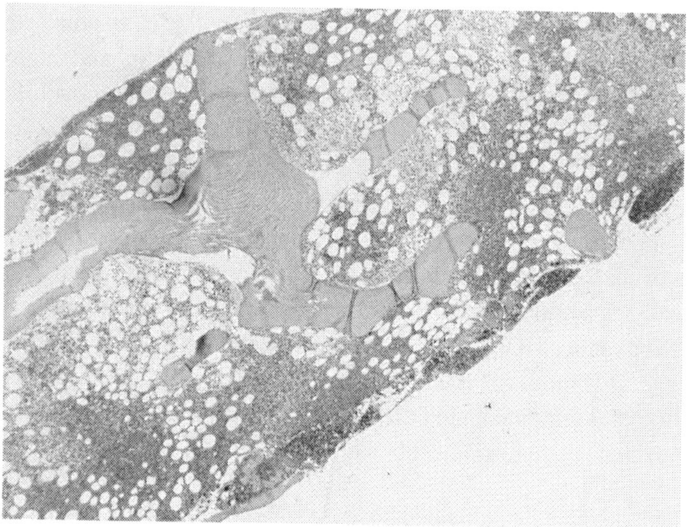

Figure 6. Mantle cell lymphoma in bone marrow. The bone marrow shows predominantly nodular pattern of infiltrate by MCL.

Most cases of MCL demonstrate a characteristic immunophenotype by flow cytometry and immunohistochemistry. By flow cytometry, the MCL cells are positive for B-cell antigens CD19, CD20, CD22, CD79a, CD79b and FMC-7, and show moderate to bright expression of surface IgM/IgD with preferential expression of lambda light chain over kappa. [8, 58-60] The expression of CD20, CD22 and FMC-7 are usually moderate and brighter compared to that of chronic lymphocytic leukemia (CLL). [58, 61, 62] FMC-7 may be negative in approximately 10% of the cases. [63] The CD19 expression may be dimmer than that of normal B-cells. [64, 65] The MCL cells characteristically show aberrant expression of CD5 and CD43, but not CD23. [60, 66, 67] However, CD5-negative and/or CD23-positive cases of MCL occur infrequently and may cause diagnostic confusion with CLL or other low grade B-cell lymphoproliferative disorder. [63, 68-70] Therefore, the CD5+/CD23- phenotype is not entirely specific for MCL and fluorescence in situ hybridization analysis for t(11;14)/IGH-CCND1 translocation is essential for confirmation of the diagnosis, especially in the peripheral blood samples. The MCL cells are usually negative for CD10, CD11c, and CD103. [60, 71,

72] CD200 is a relatively new marker that is either completely negative or dimly expressed in a subset of cells in MCL, and brightly expressed in cells of CLL. [72-74] CD200 is a useful marker for the differential diagnosis between MCL and CLL. However, occasional cases of MCL (approximately 5%) show moderately bright expression of CD200. [75] Therefore, it is important to interpret the result of CD200 expression with other markers including CD5 and CD23 for correct diagnosis. The blastoid MCL shows the typical phenotype of classic MCL (CD5+/CD23-), but more often display aberrant expression of CD10. [38, 76] Rare cases of MCL have been found to show aberrant expression of other T-cell antigens, such as CD7 and CD8. [77-79]

On tissue sections, immunohistochemical stains typically show the MCL cells positive for CD20, CD79a, PAX5, and CD5, and negative for CD23 (Figure 7). MCL are nearly always (Over 95% of cases) positive for cyclin D1 by immunohistochemical stain with the rabbit monoclonal antibody, although the staining may be heterogeneous (Figure 7). [80, 81] Cyclin D1 is the protein product of CCND1 gene, and normally undetectable in lymphocytes. The overexpression of cyclin D1 is the direct result of IGH/CCND1 translocation, and its expression in B-cells is used to confirm the diagnosis of MCL, and indicative of the presence of t(11;14)(q13;q32)/IGH-CCND1 translocation. However, cyclin D1 expression by immunohistochemical stain is not entirely specific for mantle cell lymphoma. Cyclin D1 is positive in cells of hairy cell leukemia, some cases of plasma cell myeloma, and proliferation centers of chronic lymphocytic leukemia/small lymphocytic lymphoma (CLL/SLL). [82-84] The cyclin D1 expression in hairy cell leukemia and the proliferation centers of CLL/SLL is not associated with t(11;14)(q13;q32). [85, 86] Of note, a rare case of hairy cell leukemia with IGH/CCND1 translocation has been reported. [87] CyclinD1 expression in plasma cell myeloma does not necessarily indicate the presence of t(11;14)(q13;q32), although it is always positive in plasma cell myeloma with t(11;14)(q13;q32). [88, 89] Cyclin D1 is also expressed in a small subset of CD5-negative diffuse large B-cell lymphoma (DLBCL) without translocation of the CCND1 gene locus. [90] SOX11 is a new marker that has been shown to be useful in the differential diagnosis of MCL with other low grade small B-cell lymphomas. [91] SOX11 is a neutral transcription factor normally expressed in the embryonic central nervous system, and is not expressed in normal lymphocytes. It functions as an oncogene in MCL by upregulating PAX5 and inhibits B-cell maturation and promotes angiogenesis through transcriptional regulation of PDGFA. [92, 93] SOX11 is expressed in approximately 95% cases of MCL, including cyclin D1-negative MCL [91, 94-97] The SOX11 stain is nuclear and usually intense in the majority of the MCL cells. SOX11 stain is likely to be useful in the differential diagnosis between MCL and cyclin D1-positive DLBCLs, which are negative for SOX11. [98] Although SOX11 is negative in most other small B-cell lymphomas, including CLL/SLL, follicular lymphoma, marginal zone lymphoma and all cases of plasma cell myeloma including ones with t(11;14)(q13;q32), it is not specific for MCL, and has been shown to be expressed in B-lymphoblastic leukemia/lymphoma, Burkitt lymphoma, cyclin D1 positive hairy cell leukemia and T-cell prolymphocytic leukemia. [94, 95] The indolent MCL is usually negative or dimly positive for SOX11. [22] There are several commercially available antibodies for SOX11 targeting at different epitopes, and a recent study questioned the specificity of the polyclonal antibody against SOX11 in differentiate MCL from other low grade B-cell lymphomas. [99] Therefore, the mouse monoclonal antibodies against SOX11 are recommended for clinical use.

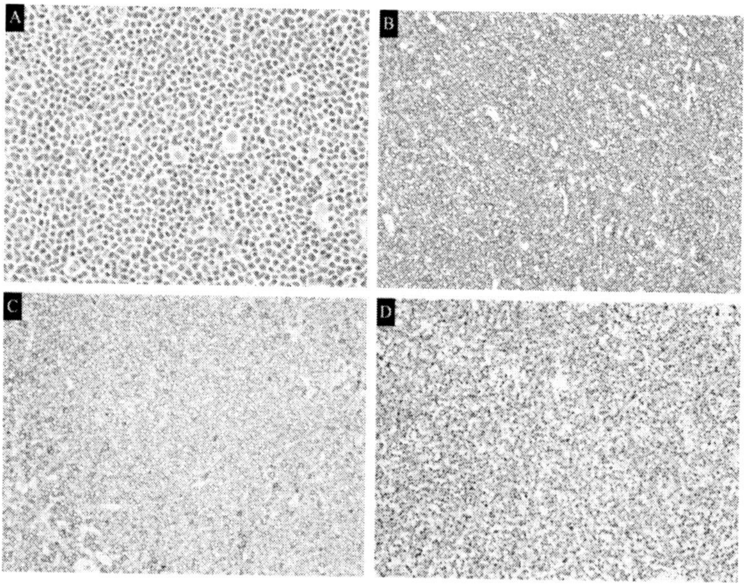


Figure 7. Mantle cell lymphoma. (A), H&E (B), CD20 (C), CD5 (D), cyclin D1.

## Mantle Cell Lymphoma *In Situ*

Mantle cell lymphoma in situ (MCLIS) is morphologically defined as presence of small numbers of cyclin D1 positive B-cells in the normal mantle zones of reactive germinal centers (Figure 8). [20, 100] The lymph nodes or extranodal lymphoid tissue show intact architecture with follicular hyperplasia. The mantle zones are not expanded, and most of the mantle cells are negative for cyclin D1. The cyclin D1 positive cells are usually present within the inner portion of mantle zones adjacent to the germinal centers. SOX11 is positive in 44% cases of MCLIS. [20] MCLIS cells are positive for IGH/CCND1 translocation. [20] MCLIS has been found to coexist with follicular lymphoma and follicular lymphoma in situ in rare cases. [101, 102] MCLIS is an incidental finding only identified by immunohistochemical stain for cyclin D1. It is important to differentiate MCLIS from MCL with mantle zone pattern and partial involvement by overt MCL in another site. In MCL with mantle zone pattern, the mantle zones are expanded and composed nearly completely of cyclin D1 and CD5 positive B-cells. In contrast to MCL with mantle zone pattern, MCLIS has a very indolent clinical course with most patients showing no progression to lymphoma. [20] Currently, it is not recommended to screen for MCLIS in reactive lymphoid tissue by immunohistochemical stain for cyclin D1. In patients diagnosed with MCLIS, a complete staging study should be performed to rule out partial involvement by an overt MCL elsewhere, and any suspicious sites should be biopsied. If no other lesions are identified through staging study, a "wait-and-see" approach is warranted.

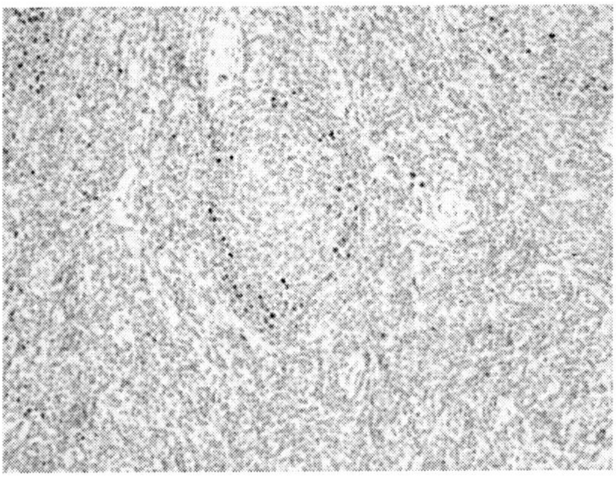

Figure 8. Mantle cell lymphoma in situ. Cyclin D1 positive cells comprise a minority of the mantle zone cells and largely confined to the inner portion of unexpanded mantle zones.

# Differential Diagnosis

The diagnosis of MCL is straightforward in most cases by demonstrating the characteristic morphology and phenotype (CD5+/CD23-), and positive immunohistochemical stain for cyclin D1 or IGH/CCND1 translocation by FISH or cytogenetic studies. Given the morphologic overlap with other B-cell lymphomas and a number of reactive conditions, it is important to keep MCL in the differential diagnosis and order appropriate studies. The accurate diagnosis of MCL is critical for patient management and prognostic evaluation.

## Reactive Lymphoid Hyperplasia

MCL with mantle zone pattern without obvious architecture effacement may be confused with reactive follicular hyperplasia and Castleman disease of the hyaline vascular type. The mantle zones of MCL with mantle zone pattern are usually thickened and diffusely positive for CD5 and cyclin D1. The mantle zones of reactive follicular hyperplasia show polarization and may have some cells positive for CD5, but are always negative for cyclin D1. Castleman disease of the hyaline vascular type typically shows thickened mantle zones surrounding variably atrophic germinal centers. The "onion skin" pattern of concentric rimming of germinal center by mantle zone cells in Castleman disease is absent in MCL with mantle zone pattern. The mantle zones in Castleman disease are also negative for CD5 and cyclin D1.

## Chronic Lymphocytic Leukemia/Small Lymphocytic Lymphoma

The differential diagnosis of MCL and CLL/SLL may be problematic in the peripheral blood sample. The cells of CLL/SLL typically show round nuclei with densely clumped "earth cracking" chromatin, while the cells of MCL usually show more irregular nuclei and mature but less condensed chromatin. However, there is significant cytological overlap between the cells of MCL and CLL/SLL. The small cell variant of MCL closely resembles CLL/SLL morphologically, and CLL/SLL with trisomy 12 usually shows cells with cleaved nuclei. [103, 104] While MCL is characterized by expression of CD5 but negative CD23, and CLL/SLL is positive for both CD5 and CD23, cases with the typical phenotype of MCL identified by flow cytometry using CD5 and CD23 also include CLL/SLL. Therefore, when tissue blocks are not available for immunohistochemical stain for cyclin D1, FISH study for IGH/CCND1 translocation is required to confirm the diagnosis of MCL even in cases with typical MCL phenotype. The new marker CD200 may improve the specificity of phenotypic diagnosis by flow cytometry. [72] In tissue sections, CLL/SLL usually shows proliferation centers composed of prolymphocytes and paraimmunoblasts, which are absent in MCL. Positive immunohistochemical stain for cyclin D1 confirms the diagnosis of MCL without the need to perform FISH study for IGH/CCND1 translocation. It should be noted that cells of the proliferation centers of CLL/SLL are positive for cyclin D1. In the so called accelerated CLL/SLL, the proliferation centers are markedly expanded and often coalesce, [105] and the pattern of immunohistochemical stain for cyclin D1 may resemble MCL. Careful attention to the cellular composition of the lymphoma cells (prolymphocytes and paraimmunoblasts in CLL/SLL) would lead one to the right track. Two new markers for immunohistochemical stain SOX11 and LEF1 are particularly useful for the differential diagnosis of MCL and CLL/SLL. [95, 98, 106] MCL is positive for SOX11 and negative for LEF1, while the reverse pattern of staining is seen in CLL/SLL.

## Monoclonal B-cell Lymphocytosis

There is no minimal level required for the diagnosis of MCL in the peripheral blood. When the numbers of circulating MCL cells are low, it is important to differentiate it from monoclonal B-cell lymphocytosis (MBL). MBL is defined as presence of $<5\text{x } 10^9$ cell/L clonal B-cells in the peripheral blood with either a CLL or non-CLL phenotype. [107] In MBL with non-CLL phenotype, some cases are positive for CD5 and negative for CD23, phenotypically indistinguishable from MCL. As MBL has an indolent clinical course, FISH study for IGH/CCND1 translocation is necessary for the correct diagnosis.

## Follicular Lymphoma

The cells of classic MCL have irregular to angulated nuclei that resemble germinal center centrocytes, hence the initial designation as "centrocytic lymphoma". Some cases of MCL have a vaguely nodular pattern which further resembles follicular lymphoma by both the growth pattern and cytology. The atypical follicles in follicular lymphoma are composed of both centrocytes and centroblasts. In contrast, the vague nodules of MCL comprise a monotonous population of centrocyte-like cells but no centroblasts. Immunohistochemical stains for germinal center markers CD10, BCL6 and MCL specific markers CD5 and cyclin D1 will reach the correct diagnosis. A subset of the blastoid/pleomorphic variants of MCL often shows aberrant expression of CD10 and BCL6, [63, 108, 109] but the expression of cyclin D1 is not expected in follicular lymphoma.

## Hairy Cell Leukemia

Hairy cell leukemia (HCL) is usually easy to diagnose due to the characteristic cytological features and immunophenotype (CD11c brightly +, CD103+, CD25+ and CD123+). [110] However, when HCL is not suspected clinically and a bone marrow biopsy is performed to evaluate cytopenia, the HCL may be misdiagnosed as MCL, as HCL cells are often rarely seen on aspirate smears and positive for both cyclin D1 and SOX11. It is important to keep HCL in the differential diagnosis of cyclin D1 positive B-cell lymphomas. If flow cytometry is not possible, immunohistochemical stain for CD5, DBA.44 and Annexin A1 should resolve the differential diagnosis. [111, 112] HCL is positive for DBA.44 and Annexin A1, and negative for CD5, while the reverse is true for MCL.

## Marginal Zone Lymphomas

There are three types of marginal zone lymphoma (MZL) recognized by the 2008 WHO classification: splenic marginal zone lymphoma, nodal marginal zone lymphoma, and extranodal marginal zone of mucosa-associated lymphoid tissue (MALT lymphoma). [17] Splenic marginal zone lymphoma may mimic the indolent MCL with lymphocytosis, splenomegaly and absence of lymphadenopathy. Splenic MZL may have variable numbers of circulating lymphoma cells that can show aberrant expression of CD5 by flow cytometry. [113] In such cases, FISH study for IGH/CCND1 translocation is required for definitive diagnosis. In tissue sections, all three forms of MZL are characterized by expansion of marginal zones surrounding reactive germinal centers. Occasionally, MCL cells may have more abundant cytoplasm mimicking marginal zones. The diagnosis can be reached with immunohistochemical stain for cyclin D1 and SOX11, which are both negative in MZL.

### B-lymphoblastic Leukemia/Lymphoma

The cells of blastoid MCL are usually small to medium-sized with fine chromatin, cytologically indistinguishable from lymphoblasts. B-lymphoblastic leukemia/lymphoma (B-ALL) cells are positive for TDT, CD34 and CD10, and negative for CD5 and cyclin D1. CD20 is typically strongly positive in MCL cells, and often negative in the cells of B-ALL. A standard panel including these antibodies is recommended in the diagnosis of blastoid MCL.

### Diffuse Large B-cell Lymphoma

The cells of pleomorphic variant of MCL often resemble lymphoma cells in diffuse large B-cell lymphoma (DLBCL). CD5 can be positive in up to 15% of DLBCL. In the absence of immunohistochemical stain for cyclin D1, the pleomorphic variant of MCL may be misdiagnosed as CD5 positive DLBCL. Therefore, it is recommended that cyclin D1 be included in the standard immunostain-panel for the diagnosis of DLBCL. A small subset of DLBCL shows aberrant expression of cyclin D1 independent of IGH/CCND1 translocation. [98] SOX11 and CD5 are most useful in this differential diagnosis, as the cyclin D1 positive DLBCLs are always negative for SOX11 and usually negative for CD5. FISH study for IGH/CCND1 translocation can also be performed on tissue sections in equivocal cases to confirm the diagnosis.

## Genetic and Molecular Features

The genetic hallmark of MCL is the t(11;14)(q13;q32) (Figure 9A) that result in fusion of immunoglobulin heavy chain enhancer to the proto-oncogene CCND1, which encodes cyclin D1. [114] This translocation results in constitutive overexpression of cyclin D1. [115, 116] Cyclin D1 is critical for cell cycle progression through the G1/S phase. [117] Cyclin D1 binds cyclin dependent kinase (CDK) 4/6 and promotes phosphorylation of the retinoblastoma protein (RB). The phosphorylation results in release of E2F transcription factor from RB, and progression through the G1/S check point into S phase of the cell cycle. The increased cyclin D1 in MCL also results in sequestration of cell cycle inhibitors such as p21/p27kip1, which further facilitate the cell cycle progression. The IGH/CCND1 translocation is present in most cases of MCL (>95%). [118, 119] Rare cases of MCL show variant translocation of CCND1 with immunoglobulin light chain gene locus. [120] There are three main breakpoints in the CCND1 gene locus: the major translocation cluster (MTC), and two minor translocation clusters (mTC1 and mTC2). [121] Approximately 30-40% CCND1 translocation in MCL involves the MTC, which is located farthest upstream of the CCND1 gene, and spans 80-100 bp. This region was originally named B-cell lymphoma/leukemia 1 region (BCL1). The minor translocation clusters are also upstream of the CCND1 gene but at a closer location relative to MTC. Approximately 5-10% cases of MCL also have deletion and mutations in the 3' UTR region of CCND1 that result in increased stability of transcript, which is associated with increased proliferation rate and poor survival. [122, 123] The IGH/CCND1 translocation can be identified by conventional karyotyping, fluorescence in situ hybridization (FISH) or PCR. Most PCR assays are designed to target the major translocation cluster region. Therefore, PCR assay only has a sensitivity of about 30-40%. In contrast, FISH study has nearly 100% sensitivity in detect CCND1 translocation due to the large region covered by the FISH probes (Figure 9B). Therefore, in situations where cytogenetic confirmation is required, FISH is the study of choice.

Rare cases of MCL are negative for IGH/CCDN1 translocation and cyclin D1 overexpression, yet show identical gene expression signature with typical MCL. [18] These cases show high expression of cyclin D2 and/or cyclin D3, with CCND2 translocation in approximately half of the cases. [18, 124, 125] Immunohistochemical stains for cyclin D2 and cyclin D3 can not be used clinically for diagnostic purpose, as these antibodies are not entirely specific and expressed in most other types of B-cell lymphomas. [126, 127] The cyclin D1-negative MCLs have been found to be uniformly positive for SOX11. [18, 95] Therefore, SOX11 is currently the best marker available for confirming the diagnosis of cyclin D1 negative MCL.

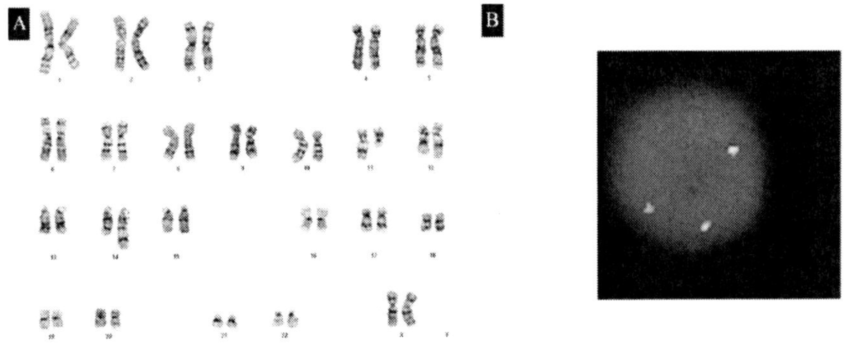

Figure 9. t(11;14)(q13;q32)/IGH-CCND1 translocation in mantle cell lymphoma. (A), metaphase karyotype of MCL with t(11;14)(q13;q32) (B), interphase FISH assay for IGH/CCND1 translocation with dual color and dual fusion probe (red signal: CCND1; green signal: IGH; yellow signal: IGH/CCND1 fusion. Courtesy of Dr. Peter Papenhausen at Cytogenetics Laboratory, Laboratory Corporation of America, Research Triangle Park, NC).

In addition to IGH/CCND1 translocation, secondary cytogenetic changes are common in MCL, including deletions of 1p, 13q and 17p, 10p alterations and 3q gains, as well as recurrent breakpoints at 1p31-32, 1p21-22, 17p13, and 1p36. [128, 129] Blastoid/pleomorphic MCL shows more karyotypic complexity, including a higher frequency of 1p and 17p deletions and 10p alterations. The rare cases of MCL with MYC gene rearrangement or amplification typically have a complex karyotype with numerous duplications and deletions of chromosomal segments in chromosomes 1p, 1q, 6p, 8p, 8q, 9p, 10p, 11q, 13q, 14q, 18p, 18q, and 22q identified by SNP array. Gains of 3q and 17p losses identified by conventional cytogenetics are associated with poor prognosis independent of proliferation index. Comparative genomic hybridization (CGH) and single nucleotide polymorphism arrays [130-133] revealed losses in 1p13.2-p31.1, 6q16.2-q27, 8p21.3, 9p13.2-p24.3, 9q13-q31.3, 11q14.3-q23.3, 13q14.13-q21.31, 13q33.1-q34, and 22q11.23-q13.33, gains involving 3q21.2-q29, 7p12.1-p22.3, 8q24.13-q24.23, and 18q21.33-q22.3, deletion of INK4A/ARF, duplication/amplification of MYC, deletion of ATM, deletion of TP53, duplication/amplification at 13q involving oncogenic microRNA, miR17-92, duplication/amplification of cyclin D1, del(1p), del(6q), dup(3q) and dup(18q). The deletion of INK4A/ARF gene locus results in decreased level of $p16^{INK4a}$, which lead to increased cyclin D1/CDK4/6 activity in promoting cell cycle progression. The deletion of ATM gene leads to impaired DNA repair and subsequent genomic instability. The deletion and mutations of TP53 result in impaired DNA repair and increased cell proliferation.

Recently, next-generation sequencing techniques with whole transcript-tome, whole genome/whole exome sequencing have been applied to MCL, and identified a number of significantly mutated genes, including NOTCH1, NOTCH2, ATM, CCND1, TP53, BIRC3, TLR2, WHSC1, MLL2, and MEF2B. [134, 135] Whole genome/exome sequencing studies also demonstrated existence of subclonal heterogeneity at the time of diagnosis and evidence of subsequent clonal evolution at the molecular level. [135]

## Prognostic Factors

MCL is an aggressive disease with the poorest survival among B-cell lymphomas (median survival of 3-5 years). [4] The blastoid variant MCL has a very aggressive clinical course with median overall survival of 14.5 months. [136] Conventional chemotherapy regimens can not cure the disease, and intense regimens including autologous or allogeneic hematopoietic stem cells transplant may offer better chance of survival. [137, 138] On the other hand, the indolent MCL with lymphocytosis, absence of lymphadenopathy, bone marrow involvement and sometime splenomegaly has a median survival of 79 months. [139] Most patients with MCL in situ do not progress to overt lymphoma, although a couple of patients with overt MCL do have MCL in situ when previous tissues are examined. [20] The choice of treatment for patients is dependent on stratifying the patients based on their individual risk for disease progression and relapse.

The most important prognostic factor on histology is the proliferation rate based on either the numbers of mitotic figures under high power fields or proliferation index assessed by immunohistochemical stain for Ki-67. A high mitotic figures >10-37.5/15 hfp, or $>50/mm^2$ or high percentage of Ki-67 positive lymphoma cells >40% or >60% is associated with poor prognosis. [4, 41, 140-142] Gene expression profiling studies also showed that a proliferation signature composed of 20 genes is most important in predicting prognosis in MCL. [143, 144] Several other histologically and genetic features have been found to be associated with adverse prognosis, and are likely associated with the proliferation index: blastoid/pleomorphic morphology, TP53 abnormalities, and trisomy 12. [130-132, 141, 145, 146] Chromosomal 3q gains and 9q losses are associated with adverse prognosis independent of the gene expression-based proliferation signature. [133] The importance of growth pattern of MCL in predicting prognosis is less clear. [14, 43, 147]

The International Prognostic Index (IPI) designed for diffuse large B-cell lymphoma is less useful in MCL, and Mantle Cell International Prognostic Index (MIPI) was proposed. [148] MIPI stratifies patients into low risk (median OS not reached), intermediate risk (median OS of 51 months), and high risk groups (median OS of 29 months) based on 4 independent prognostic factors: age, performance status, lactate dehydrogenase (LDH), and leukocyte count.

The proliferation index by Ki-67 was shown to be important and provided strong additional prognostic relevance. [148] The MIPI has been widely used in clinical practice nowadays.

## Conclusion

Although not a diagnostic challenge in most cases, MCL has unusual variants that may cause problems in reaching the correct diagnosis. MCL should always be in the differential diagnosis when diagnosing small and large B-cell lymphomas, and appropriate ancillary studies should be ordered to confirm the diagnosis. It is important for the pathologist to document in the pathology report the presence of aggressive variants (blastoid and pleomorphic MCL) and the proliferation rate either by counting the mitotic figures or immunohistochemical stain for Ki-67. The clinician should be aware of the clinical features of indolent MCL and MCL in situ to avoid overtreatment of these patients.

The addition of new antibodies for MCL continues to improve the sensitivity and specificity of flow cytometry and immunohistochemical stain for the diagnosis of MCL. Although currently still not widely in use clinically, the gene expression profiling and new molecular cytogenetic techniques, such as next-generation sequencing not only will shed light on the molecular mechanism for lymphomagenesis in MCL but also likely generate candidate targets for diagnostic use and the development of reagents for targeted therapy.

# References


[1] Lennert, K., Stein, H. & Kaiserling, E. Cytological and functional criteria for the classification of malignant lymphomata. *The British journal of cancer. Supplement* 2, 29-43 (1975).

[2] Weisenburger, D. D., Kim, H. & Rappaport, H. Mantle-zone lymphoma: a follicular variant of intermediate lymphocytic lymphoma. *Cancer* 49, 1429-1438 (1982).

[3] Jaffe, E. S., Bookman, M. A. & Longo, D. L. Lymphocytic lymphoma of intermediate differentiation--mantle zone lymphoma: a distinct subtype of B-cell lymphoma. *Human pathology* 18, 877-880 (1987).

[4] Swerdlow, S. H. et al. Centrocytic lymphoma: a distinct clinicopathologic and immunologic entity. A multiparameter study of 18 cases at diagnosis and relapse. *The American journal of pathology* 113, 181-197 (1983).

[5] Stein, H., Gerdes, J. & Mason, D. Y. The normal and malignant germinal centre. *Clinics in haematology* 11, 531-559 (1982).

[6] Stein, H., Lennert, K., Feller, A. C. & Mason, D. Y. Immunohistological analysis of human lymphoma: correlation of histological and immunological categories. *Advances in cancer research* 42, 67-147 (1984).

[7] Frizzera, G., Sakurai, M., Notohara, K. & Konishi, H. t(11;14) (q13;q32) in B-cell lymphomas (intermediately differentiated lymphocytic and follicular). A report of four cases. *American journal of clinical pathology* 95, 684-691 (1991).

[8] Leroux, D. et al. Non-Hodgkin's lymphomas with t(11;14)(q13;q32): a subset of mantle zone/intermediate lymphocytic lymphoma? *British journal of haematology* 77, 346-353 (1991).

[9] Medeiros, L. J., Van Krieken, J. H., Jaffe, E. S. & Raffeld, M. Association of bcl-1 rearrangements with lymphocytic lymphoma of intermediate differentiation. *Blood* 76, 2086-2090 (1990).

[10] Rosenberg, C. L. et al. PRAD1, a candidate BCL1 oncogene: mapping and expression in centrocytic lymphoma. *Proceedings of the National Academy of Sciences of the United States of America* 88, 9638-9642 (1991).

[11] Vandenberghe, E. et al. Translocation (11;14): a cytogenetic anomaly associated with B-cell lymphomas of non-follicle centre cell lineage.

*The Journal of pathology* 163, 13-18, doi:10.1002/path.1711630104 (1991).

[12] Weisenburger, D. D., Sanger, W. G., Armitage, J. O. & Purtilo, D. T. Intermediate lymphocytic lymphoma: immunophenotypic and cytogenetic findings. *Blood* 69, 1617-1621 (1987).

[13] Williams, M. E., Westermann, C. D. & Swerdlow, S. H. Genotypic characterization of centrocytic lymphoma: frequent rearrangement of the chromosome 11 bcl-1 locus. *Blood* 76, 1387-1391 (1990).

[14] Majlis, A., Pugh, W. C., Rodriguez, M. A., Benedict, W. F. & Cabanillas, F. Mantle cell lymphoma: correlation of clinical outcome and biologic features with three histologic variants. *Journal of clinical oncology : official journal of the American Society of Clinical Oncology* 15, 1664-1671 (1997).

[15] Banks, P. M. et al. Mantle cell lymphoma. A proposal for unification of morphologic, immunologic, and molecular data. *The American journal of surgical pathology* 16, 637-640 (1992).

[16] Harris, N. L. et al. A revised European-American classification of lymphoid neoplasms: a proposal from the International Lymphoma Study Group. *Blood* 84, 1361-1392 (1994).

[17] Swerdlow SH, C. E., Harris NL, Jaffe ES, Pileri SA, Stein H. *WHO classification of tumours of haematopoietic and lymphoid tissues.* (IARC,Lyon, 2008).

[18] Fu, K. et al. Cyclin D1-negative mantle cell lymphoma: a clinicopathologic study based on gene expression profiling. *Blood* 106, 4315-4321, doi:10.1182/blood-2005-04-1753 (2005).

[19] Furtado, M. & Rule, S. Indolent mantle cell lymphoma. *Haematologica* 96, 1086-1088, doi:10.3324/haematol.2011.047357 (2011).

[20] Carvajal-Cuenca, A. et al. In situ mantle cell lymphoma: clinical implications of an incidental finding with indolent clinical behavior. *Haematologica* 97, 270-278, doi:10.3324/haematol.2011.052621 (2012).

[21] Setoodeh, R. et al. Double-hit mantle cell lymphoma with MYC gene rearrangement or amplification: a report of four cases and review of the literature. *International journal of clinical and experimental pathology* 6, 155-167 (2013).

[22] Ondrejka, S. L., Lai, R., Smith, S. D. & Hsi, E. D. Indolent mantle cell leukemia: a clinicopathological variant characterized by isolated lymphocytosis, interstitial bone marrow involvement, kappa light chain

restriction, and good prognosis. *Haematologica* 96, 1121-1127, doi:10.3324/haematol.2010.036277 (2011).

[23] Hao, S. et al. Mantle cell lymphoma with 8q24 chromosomal abnormalities: a report of 5 cases with blastoid features. *Modern pathology : an official journal of the United States and Canadian Academy of Pathology, Inc* 15, 1266-1272, doi:10.1097/01.MP.0000037310.82136.99 (2002).

[24] A clinical evaluation of the International Lymphoma Study Group classification of non-Hodgkin's lymphoma. The Non-Hodgkin's Lymphoma Classification Project. *Blood* 89, 3909-3918 (1997).

[25] Zhou, Y. et al. Incidence trends of mantle cell lymphoma in the United States between 1992 and 2004. *Cancer* 113, 791-798, doi:10.1002/cncr.23608 (2008).

[26] Smedby, K. E. & Hjalgrim, H. Epidemiology and etiology of mantle cell lymphoma and other non-Hodgkin lymphoma subtypes. *Seminars in cancer biology* 21, 293-298, doi:10.1016/j.semcancer.2011.09.010 (2011).

[27] Ferrer, A. et al. Leukemic involvement is a common feature in mantle cell lymphoma. *Cancer* 109, 2473-2480, doi:10.1002/cncr.22715 (2007).

[28] Salar, A. et al. Gastrointestinal involvement in mantle cell lymphoma: a prospective clinic, endoscopic, and pathologic study. *The American journal of surgical pathology* 30, 1274-1280, doi:10.1097/01.pas.0000208899.15859.cb (2006).

[29] Cornes, J. S. Multiple lymphomatous polyposis of the gastrointestinal tract. *Cancer* 14, 249-257 (1961).

[30] Kodama, T. et al. Lymphomatous polyposis of the gastrointestinal tract, including mantle cell lymphoma, follicular lymphoma and mucosa-associated lymphoid tissue lymphoma. *Histopathology* 47, 467-478, doi:10.1111/j.1365-2559.2005.02225.x (2005).

[31] Misdraji, J., Harris, N. L., Hasserjian, R. P., Lauwers, G. Y. & Ferry, J. A. Primary follicular lymphoma of the gastrointestinal tract. *The American journal of surgical pathology* 35, 1255-1263, doi:10.1097/PAS.0b013e318224e661 (2011).

[32] Schmatz, A. I. et al. Primary follicular lymphoma of the duodenum is a distinct mucosal/submucosal variant of follicular lymphoma: a retrospective study of 63 cases. *Journal of clinical oncology : official journal of the American Society of Clinical Oncology* 29, 1445-1451, doi:10.1200/JCO.2010.32.9193 (2011).

[33] Shia, J. et al. Primary follicular lymphoma of the gastrointestinal tract: a clinical and pathologic study of 26 cases. *The American journal of surgical pathology* 26, 216-224 (2002).
[34] Takata, K. et al. Primary gastrointestinal follicular lymphoma involving the duodenal second portion is a distinct entity: a multicenter, retrospective analysis in Japan. *Cancer science* 102, 1532-1536, doi:10.1111/j.1349-7006.2011.01980.x (2011).
[35] Yoshino, T. et al. Increased incidence of follicular lymphoma in the duodenum. *The American journal of surgical pathology* 24, 688-693 (2000).
[36] Campo, E., Raffeld, M. & Jaffe, E. S. Mantle-cell lymphoma. *Seminars in hematology* 36, 115-127 (1999).
[37] Klapper, W. Histopathology of mantle cell lymphoma. *Seminars in hematology* 48, 148-154, doi:10.1053/j.seminhematol.2011.03.006 (2011).
[38] Lardelli, P., Bookman, M. A., Sundeen, J., Longo, D. L. & Jaffe, E. S. Lymphocytic lymphoma of intermediate differentiation. Morphologic and immunophenotypic spectrum and clinical correlations. *The American journal of surgical pathology* 14, 752-763 (1990).
[39] Tolksdorf, G., Stein, H. & Lennert, K. Morphological and immunological definition of a malignant lymphoma derived from germinal-centre cells with cleaved nuclei (centrocytes). *British journal of cancer* 41, 168-182 (1980).
[40] Young, K. H. et al. Mantle cell lymphoma with plasma cell differentiation. *The American journal of surgical pathology* 30, 954-961 (2006).
[41] Tiemann, M. et al. Histopathology, cell proliferation indices and clinical outcome in 304 patients with mantle cell lymphoma (MCL): a clinicopathological study from the European MCL Network. *British journal of haematology* 131, 29-38, doi:10.1111/j.1365-2141.2005.05716.x (2005).
[42] Kimura, Y. et al. Small cell variant of mantle cell lymphoma is an indolent lymphoma characterized by bone marrow involvement, splenomegaly, and a low Ki-67 index. *Cancer science* 102, 1734-1741, doi:10.1111/j.1349-7006.2011.01988.x (2011).
[43] Norton, A. J. et al. Mantle cell lymphoma: natural history defined in a serially biopsied population over a 20-year period. *Annals of oncology : official journal of the European Society for Medical Oncology / ESMO* 6, 249-256 (1995).

[44] Vogt, N. & Klapper, W. Variability in morphology and cell proliferation in sequential biopsies of mantle cell lymphoma at diagnosis and relapse: clinical correlation and insights into disease progression. *Histopathology* 62, 334-342, doi:10.1111/his.12009 (2013).
[45] Kansal, R., Ross, C. W., Singleton, T. P., Finn, W. G. & Schnitzer, B. Histopathologic features of splenic small B-cell lymphomas. A study of 42 cases with a definitive diagnosis by the World Health Organization classification. *American journal of clinical pathology* 120, 335-347, doi:10.1309/HWG0-84N3-F3LR-J8XB (2003).
[46] Piris, M. A. et al. A marginal zone pattern may be found in different varieties of non-Hodgkin's lymphoma: the morphology and immunohistology of splenic involvement by B-cell lymphomas simulating splenic marginal zone lymphoma. *Histopathology* 33, 230-239 (1998).
[47] Chan, J. K. Gastrointestinal lymphomas: an overview with emphasis on new findings and diagnostic problems. *Seminars in diagnostic pathology* 13, 260-296 (1996).
[48] Romaguera, J. E. et al. Frequency of gastrointestinal involvement and its clinical significance in mantle cell lymphoma. *Cancer* 97, 586-591, doi:10.1002/cncr.11096 (2003).
[49] Singleton, T. P., Anderson, M. M., Ross, C. W. & Schnitzer, B. Leukemic phase of mantle cell lymphoma, blastoid variant. *American journal of clinical pathology* 111, 495-500 (1999).
[50] van der Velden, V. H. et al. B-cell prolymphocytic leukemia: a specific subgroup of mantle cell lymphoma. *Blood* 124, 412-419, doi:10.1182/blood-2013-10-533869 (2014).
[51] Rahman, K. et al. Morphological spectrum of leukemic mantle cell lymphoma. *Indian journal of pathology & microbiology* 55, 66-71, doi:10.4103/0377-4929.94860 (2012).
[52] Ruchlemer, R. et al. B-prolymphocytic leukaemia with t(11;14) revisited: a splenomegalic form of mantle cell lymphoma evolving with leukaemia. *British journal of haematology* 125, 330-336, doi:10.1111/j.1365-2141.2004.04913.x (2004).
[53] Wong, K. F., So, C. C. & Chan, J. K. Nucleolated variant of mantle cell lymphoma with leukemic manifestations mimicking prolymphocytic leukemia. *American journal of clinical pathology* 117, 246-251, doi:10.1309/4LTE-JHNC-C8RC-FGWL (2002).
[54] Schlette, E. et al. Mature B-cell leukemias with more than 55% prolymphocytes. A heterogeneous group that includes an unusual

variant of mantle cell lymphoma. *American journal of clinical pathology* 115, 571-581, doi:10.1309/PPK0-TJUK-1UAR-3194 (2001).

[55] Cohen, P. L., Kurtin, P. J., Donovan, K. A. & Hanson, C. A. Bone marrow and peripheral blood involvement in mantle cell lymphoma. *British journal of haematology* 101, 302-310 (1998).

[56] Wasman, J., Rosenthal, N. S. & Farhi, D. C. Mantle cell lymphoma. Morphologic findings in bone marrow involvement. *American journal of clinical pathology* 106, 196-200 (1996).

[57] Viswanatha, D. S. et al. Blastic mantle cell leukemia: an unusual presentation of blastic mantle cell lymphoma. *Modern pathology : an official journal of the United States and Canadian Academy of Pathology, Inc* 13, 825-833, doi:10.1038/modpathol.3880144 (2000).

[58] D'Arena, G. et al. Quantitative flow cytometry for the differential diagnosis of leukemic B-cell chronic lymphoproliferative disorders. *American journal of hematology* 64, 275-281 (2000).

[59] Bell, P. B., Rooney, N. & Bosanquet, A. G. CD79a detected by ZL7.4 separates chronic lymphocytic leukemia from mantle cell lymphoma in the leukemic phase. *Cytometry* 38, 102-105 (1999).

[60] Weisenburger, D. D. & Armitage, J. O. Mantle cell lymphoma-- an entity comes of age. *Blood* 87, 4483-4494 (1996).

[61] Cossman, J., Neckers, L. M., Hsu, S., Longo, D. & Jaffe, E. S. Low-grade lymphomas. Expression of developmentally regulated B-cell antigens. *The American journal of pathology* 115, 117-124 (1984).

[62] Garcia, D. P., Rooney, M. T., Ahmad, E. & Davis, B. H. Diagnostic usefulness of CD23 and FMC-7 antigen expression patterns in B-cell lymphoma classification. *American journal of clinical pathology* 115, 258-265, doi:10.1309/VWTK-XYT5-D0DK-06HQ (2001).

[63] Gao, J., Peterson, L., Nelson, B., Goolsby, C. & Chen, Y. H. Immunophenotypic variations in mantle cell lymphoma. *American journal of clinical pathology* 132, 699-706, doi:10.1309/AJCPV8LN5ENMZOVY (2009).

[64] Ginaldi, L. et al. Levels of expression of CD19 and CD20 in chronic B cell leukaemias. *Journal of clinical pathology* 51, 364-369 (1998).

[65] Yang, W. et al. Diminished expression of CD19 in B-cell lymphomas. *Cytometry. Part B, Clinical cytometry* 63, 28-35, doi:10.1002/cyto.b.20030 (2005).

[66] Ahmad, E., Garcia, D. & Davis, B. H. Clinical utility of CD23 and FMC7 antigen coexistent expression in B-cell lymphoproliferative disorder subclassification. *Cytometry* 50, 1-7 (2002).

[67] Samaha, H. et al. Mantle cell lymphoma: a retrospective study of 121 cases. *Leukemia* 12, 1281-1287 (1998).

[68] Matutes, E. et al. The leukemic presentation of mantle-cell lymphoma: disease features and prognostic factors in 58 patients. *Leukemia & lymphoma* 45, 2007-2015, doi:10.1080/10428190410001723331 (2004).

[69] Kelemen, K. et al. CD23+ mantle cell lymphoma: a clinical pathologic entity associated with superior outcome compared with CD23- disease. *American journal of clinical pathology* 130, 166-177, doi:10.1309/R94MAFJY5EA4A8C3 (2008).

[70] Ho, A. K. et al. Small B-cell neoplasms with typical mantle cell lymphoma immunophenotypes often include chronic lymphocytic leukemias. *American journal of clinical pathology* 131, 27-32, doi:10.1309/AJCPPAG4VR4IPGHZ (2009).

[71] Takeshita, M. et al. Clinicopathologic, enzyme and histochemical studies of centrocytic (mantle cell) lymphoma: comparison with other types of low-grade B cell lymphoma based on the updated Kiel classification. *Acta pathologica japonica* 43, 244-252 (1993).

[72] Palumbo, G. A. et al. CD200 expression may help in differential diagnosis between mantle cell lymphoma and B-cell chronic lymphocytic leukemia. *Leukemia research* 33, 1212-1216, doi:10.1016/j.leukres.2009.01.017 (2009).

[73] Alapat, D. et al. Diagnostic usefulness and prognostic impact of CD200 expression in lymphoid malignancies and plasma cell myeloma. *American journal of clinical pathology* 137, 93-100, doi:10.1309/AJCP59UORCYZEVQO (2012).

[74] Sandes, A. F. et al. CD200 has an important role in the differential diagnosis of mature B-cell neoplasms by multiparameter flow cytometry. *Cytometry. Part B, Clinical cytometry* 86, 98-105, doi:10.1002/cyto.b.21128 (2014).

[75] Challagundla, P., Medeiros, L. J., Kanagal-Shamanna, R., Miranda, R. N. & Jorgensen, J. L. Differential expression of CD200 in B-cell neoplasms by flow cytometry can assist in diagnosis, subclassification, and bone marrow staging. *American journal of clinical pathology* 142, 837-844, doi:10.1309/AJCPBV9ELXC0ECVL (2014).

[76] Dunphy, C. H., Wheaton, S. E. & Perkins, S. L. CD23 expression in transformed small lymphocytic lymphomas/chronic lymphocytic leukemias and blastic transformations of mantle cell lymphoma. *Modern pathology : an official journal of the United States and Canadian Academy of Pathology, Inc* 10, 818-822 (1997).

[77] Hoffman, D. G., Tucker, S. J., Emmanoulides, C., Rosen, P. A. & Naeim, F. CD8-positive mantle cell lymphoma: a report of two cases. *American journal of clinical pathology* 109, 689-694 (1998).

[78] Schroers, R. et al. Immunophenotypic and genetic characterization of a CD8 positive mantle cell lymphoma in a patient with concomitant Mycosis fungoides. *European journal of haematology* 75, 78-84, doi:10.1111/j.1600-0609.2005.00432.x (2005).

[79] Kaleem, Z., White, G. & Zutter, M. M. Aberrant expression of T-cell-associated antigens on B-cell non-Hodgkin lymphomas. *American journal of clinical pathology* 115, 396-403, doi:10.1309/EHMY-7WU1-UYE7-EE99 (2001).

[80] Cheuk, W., Wong, K. O., Wong, C. S. & Chan, J. K. Consistent immunostaining for cyclin D1 can be achieved on a routine basis using a newly available rabbit monoclonal antibody. *The American journal of surgical pathology* 28, 801-807 (2004).

[81] Pruneri, G. et al. SP4, a novel anti-cyclin D1 rabbit monoclonal antibody, is a highly sensitive probe for identifying mantle cell lymphomas bearing the t(11;14)(q13;q32) translocation. *Applied immunohistochemistry & molecular morphology : AIMM / official publication of the Society for Applied Immunohistochemistry* 13, 318-322 (2005).

[82] Athanasiou, E. et al. Cyclin D1 overexpression in multiple myeloma. A morphologic, immunohistochemical, and in situ hybridization study of 71 paraffin-embedded bone marrow biopsy specimens. *American journal of clinical pathology* 116, 535-542, doi:10.1309/BVT4-YP41-LCV2-5GT0 (2001).

[83] Miranda, R. N. et al. Immunohistochemical detection of cyclin D1 using optimized conditions is highly specific for mantle cell lymphoma and hairy cell leukemia. *Modern pathology : an official journal of the United States and Canadian Academy of Pathology, Inc* 13, 1308-1314, doi:10.1038/modpathol.3880239 (2000).

[84] O'Malley, D. P., Vance, G. H. & Orazi, A. Chronic lymphocytic leukemia/small lymphocytic lymphoma with trisomy 12 and focal cyclin d1 expression: a potential diagnostic pitfall. *Archives of pathology & laboratory medicine* 129, 92-95, doi:10.1043/1543-2165(2005)129<92:CLSLLW>2.0.CO;2 (2005).

[85] Gradowski, J. F. et al. Chronic lymphocytic leukemia/small lymphocytic lymphoma with cyclin D1 positive proliferation centers do not have CCND1 translocations or gains and lack SOX11 expression.

*American journal of clinical pathology* 138, 132-139, doi:10.1309/AJCPIVKZRMPF93ET (2012).

[86] de Boer, C. J. et al. Involvement of the CCND1 gene in hairy cell leukemia. *Annals of oncology : official journal of the European Society for Medical Oncology / ESMO* 7, 251-256 (1996).

[87] Chen, D. et al. A case of hairy cell leukemia with CCND1-IGH@ translocation: indolent non-nodal mantle cell lymphoma revisited. *The American journal of surgical pathology* 35, 1080-1084, doi:10.1097/PAS.0b013e31821ddaec (2011).

[88] Hoyer, J. D. et al. The (11;14)(q13;q32) translocation in multiple myeloma. A morphologic and immunohistochemical study. *American journal of clinical pathology* 113, 831-837, doi:10.1309/4W8E-8F4K-BHUP-UBE7 (2000).

[89] Dunphy, C. H., Nies, M. K. & Gabriel, D. A. Correlation of plasma cell percentages by CD138 immunohistochemistry, cyclin D1 status, and CD56 expression with clinical parameters and overall survival in plasma cell myeloma. *Applied immunohistochemistry & molecular morphology: AIMM / official publication of the Society for Applied Immunohistochemistry* 15, 248-254, doi:10.1097/01.pai.0000213136.93912.84 (2007).

[90] Vela-Chavez, T. et al. Cyclin D1 positive diffuse large B-cell lymphoma is a post-germinal center-type lymphoma without alterations in the CCND1 gene locus. *Leukemia & lymphoma* 52, 458-466, doi:10.3109/10428194.2010.540361 (2011).

[91] Ek, S., Dictor, M., Jerkeman, M., Jirstrom, K. & Borrebaeck, C. A. Nuclear expression of the non B-cell lineage Sox11 transcription factor identifies mantle cell lymphoma. *Blood* 111, 800-805, doi:10.1182/blood-2007-06-093401 (2008).

[92] Vegliante, M. C. et al. SOX11 regulates PAX5 expression and blocks terminal B-cell differentiation in aggressive mantle cell lymphoma. *Blood* 121, 2175-2185, doi:10.1182/blood-2012-06-438937 (2013).

[93] Palomero, J. et al. SOX11 promotes tumor angiogenesis through transcriptional regulation of PDGFA in mantle cell lymphoma. *Blood* 124, 2235-2247, doi:10.1182/blood-2014-04-569566 (2014).

[94] Chen, Y. H., Gao, J., Fan, G. & Peterson, L. C. Nuclear expression of sox11 is highly associated with mantle cell lymphoma but is independent of t(11;14)(q13;q32) in non-mantle cell B-cell neoplasms. *Modern pathology : an official journal of the United States and*

*Canadian Academy of Pathology, Inc* 23, 105-112, doi:10.1038/modpathol.2009.140 (2010).

[95] Mozos, A. et al. SOX11 expression is highly specific for mantle cell lymphoma and identifies the cyclin D1-negative subtype. *Haematologica* 94, 1555-1562, doi:10.3324/haematol.2009.010264 (2009).

[96] Dictor, M. et al. Strong lymphoid nuclear expression of SOX11 transcription factor defines lymphoblastic neoplasms, mantle cell lymphoma and Burkitt's lymphoma. *Haematologica* 94, 1563-1568, doi:10.3324/haematol.2009.008474 (2009).

[97] Meggendorfer, M., Kern, W., Haferlach, C., Haferlach, T. & Schnittger, S. SOX11 overexpression is a specific marker for mantle cell lymphoma and correlates with t(11;14) translocation, CCND1 expression and an adverse prognosis. *Leukemia* 27, 2388-2391, doi:10.1038/leu.2013.141 (2013).

[98] Hsiao, S. C. et al. SOX11 is useful in differentiating cyclin D1-positive diffuse large B-cell lymphoma from mantle cell lymphoma. *Histopathology* 61, 685-693, doi:10.1111/j.1365-2559.2012.04260.x (2012).

[99] Zhang, L. N. et al. Polyclonal antibody targeting SOX11 cannot differentiate mantle cell lymphoma from B-cell non-Hodgkin lymphomas. *American journal of clinical pathology* 140, 795-800, doi:10.1309/AJCPEBOUJ7GVYVLG (2013).

[100] Fend, F. et al. Early lesions in lymphoid neoplasia: Conclusions based on the Workshop of the XV. Meeting of the European Association of Hematopathology and the Society of Hematopathology, in Uppsala, Sweden. *Journal of hematopathology* 5, doi:10.1007/s12308-012-0148-6 (2012).

[101] Roullet, M. R. et al. Coexisting follicular and mantle cell lymphoma with each having an in situ component: A novel, curious, and complex consultation case of coincidental, composite, colonizing lymphoma. *American journal of clinical pathology* 133, 584-591, doi:10.1309/AJCP5RT4MRSDGKSX (2010).

[102] Taverna, J. et al. A rare presentation of in situ mantle cell lymphoma and follicular lymphoma: a case report and review of the literature. *Case reports in hematology* 2014, 145129, doi:10.1155/2014/145129 (2014).

[103] Matutes, E. et al. Trisomy 12 defines a group of CLL with atypical morphology: correlation between cytogenetic, clinical and laboratory

features in 544 patients. *British journal of haematology* 92, 382-388 (1996).

[104] Frater, J. L. et al. Typical and atypical chronic lymphocytic leukemia differ clinically and immunophenotypically. *American journal of clinical pathology* 116, 655-664, doi:10.1309/7Q1J-1AA8-DU4Q-PVLQ (2001).

[105] Gine, E. et al. Expanded and highly active proliferation centers identify a histological subtype of chronic lymphocytic leukemia ("accelerated" chronic lymphocytic leukemia) with aggressive clinical behavior. *Haematologica* 95, 1526-1533, doi:10.3324/haematol.2010.022277 (2010).

[106] Tandon, B. et al. Nuclear overexpression of lymphoid-enhancer-binding factor 1 identifies chronic lymphocytic leukemia/small lymphocytic lymphoma in small B-cell lymphomas. *Modern pathology : an official journal of the United States and Canadian Academy of Pathology, Inc* 24, 1433-1443, doi:10.1038/modpathol.2011.103 (2011).

[107] Parikh, S. A., Kay, N. E. & Shanafelt, T. D. Monoclonal B-cell lymphocytosis: update on diagnosis, clinical outcome, and counseling. *Clinical advances in hematology & oncology : H&O* 11, 720-729 (2013).

[108] Camacho, F. I. et al. Aberrant Bcl6 protein expression in mantle cell lymphoma. *The American journal of surgical pathology* 28, 1051-1056 (2004).

[109] Gualco, G., Weiss, L. M., Harrington, W. J., Jr. & Bacchi, C. E. BCL6, MUM1, and CD10 expression in mantle cell lymphoma. *Applied immunohistochemistry & molecular morphology : AIMM / official publication of the Society for Applied Immunohistochemistry* 18, 103-108, doi:10.1097/PAI.0b013e3181bb9edf (2010).

[110] Shao, H. et al. Distinguishing hairy cell leukemia variant from hairy cell leukemia: development and validation of diagnostic criteria. *Leukemia research* 37, 401-409, doi:10.1016/j.leukres.2012.11.021 (2013).

[111] Went, P. T. et al. High specificity of combined TRAP and DBA.44 expression for hairy cell leukemia. *The American journal of surgical pathology* 29, 474-478 (2005).

[112] Toth-Liptak, J. et al. A Comprehensive Immunophenotypic Marker Analysis of Hairy Cell Leukemia in Paraffin-Embedded Bone Marrow Trephine Biopsies-A Tissue Microarray Study. *Pathology oncology research : POR*, doi:10.1007/s12253-014-9807-5 (2014).

[113] Kojima, M. et al. Characteristics of CD5-positive splenic marginal zone lymphoma with leukemic manifestation ; clinical, flow cytometry, and histopathological findings of 11 cases. *Journal of clinical and experimental hematopathology : JCEH* 50, 107-112 (2010).

[114] Bertoni, F., Rinaldi, A., Zucca, E. & Cavalli, F. Update on the molecular biology of mantle cell lymphoma. *Hematological oncology* 24, 22-27, doi:10.1002/hon.767 (2006).

[115] de Boer, C. J., van Krieken, J. H., Kluin-Nelemans, H. C., Kluin, P. M. & Schuuring, E. Cyclin D1 messenger RNA overexpression as a marker for mantle cell lymphoma. *Oncogene* 10, 1833-1840 (1995).

[116] Seto, M. et al. Gene rearrangement and overexpression of PRAD1 in lymphoid malignancy with t(11;14)(q13;q32) translocation. *Oncogene* 7, 1401-1406 (1992).

[117] Kim, J. K. & Diehl, J. A. Nuclear cyclin D1: an oncogenic driver in human cancer. *Journal of cellular physiology* 220, 292-296, doi:10.1002/jcp.21791 (2009).

[118] Jares, P., Colomer, D. & Campo, E. Genetic and molecular pathogenesis of mantle cell lymphoma: perspectives for new targeted therapeutics. *Nature reviews. Cancer* 7, 750-762, doi:10.1038/nrc2230 (2007).

[119] Perez-Galan, P., Dreyling, M. & Wiestner, A. Mantle cell lymphoma: biology, pathogenesis, and the molecular basis of treatment in the genomic era. *Blood* 117, 26-38, doi:10.1182/blood-2010-04-189977 (2011).

[120] Komatsu, H. et al. A variant chromosome translocation at 11q13 identifying PRAD1/cyclin D1 as the BCL-1 gene. *Blood* 84, 1226-1231 (1994).

[121] Fernandez, V., Hartmann, E., Ott, G., Campo, E. & Rosenwald, A. Pathogenesis of mantle-cell lymphoma: all oncogenic roads lead to dysregulation of cell cycle and DNA damage response pathways. *Journal of clinical oncology : official journal of the American Society of Clinical Oncology* 23, 6364-6369, doi:10.1200/JCO.2005.05.019 (2005).

[122] Slotta-Huspenina, J. et al. The impact of cyclin D1 mRNA isoforms, morphology and p53 in mantle cell lymphoma: p53 alterations and blastoid morphology are strong predictors of a high proliferation index. *Haematologica* 97, 1422-1430, doi:10.3324/haematol.2011.055715 (2012).

[123] Wiestner, A. et al. Point mutations and genomic deletions in CCND1 create stable truncated cyclin D1 mRNAs that are associated with

increased proliferation rate and shorter survival. *Blood* 109, 4599-4606, doi:10.1182/blood-2006-08-039859 (2007).

[124] Wlodarska, I. et al. Translocations targeting CCND2, CCND3, and MYCN do occur in t(11;14)-negative mantle cell lymphomas. *Blood* 111, 5683-5690, doi:10.1182/blood-2007-10-118794 (2008).

[125] Salaverria, I. et al. CCND2 rearrangements are the most frequent genetic events in cyclin D1(-) mantle cell lymphoma. *Blood* 121, 1394-1402, doi:10.1182/blood-2012-08-452284 (2013).

[126] Quintanilla-Martinez, L. et al. Differential diagnosis of cyclin D2+ mantle cell lymphoma based on fluorescence in situ hybridization and quantitative real-time-PCR. *Haematologica* 94, 1595-1598, doi:10.3324/haematol.2009.010173 (2009).

[127] Metcalf, R. A. et al. Characterization of D-cyclin proteins in hematolymphoid neoplasms: lack of specificity of cyclin-D2 and D3 expression in lymphoma subtypes. *Modern pathology : an official journal of the United States and Canadian Academy of Pathology, Inc* 23, 420-433, doi:10.1038/modpathol.2009.173 (2010).

[128] Au, W. Y. et al. Cytogenetic analysis in mantle cell lymphoma: a review of 214 cases. *Leukemia & lymphoma* 43, 783-791, doi:10.1080/10428190290016890 (2002).

[129] Espinet, B. et al. Incidence and prognostic impact of secondary cytogenetic aberrations in a series of 145 patients with mantle cell lymphoma. *Genes, chromosomes & cancer* 49, 439-451, doi:10.1002/gcc.20754 (2010).

[130] Royo, C. et al. The complex landscape of genetic alterations in mantle cell lymphoma. *Seminars in cancer biology* 21, 322-334, doi:10.1016/j.semcancer.2011.09.007 (2011).

[131] Bea, S. et al. Uniparental disomies, homozygous deletions, amplifications, and target genes in mantle cell lymphoma revealed by integrative high-resolution whole-genome profiling. *Blood* 113, 3059-3069, doi:10.1182/blood-2008-07-170183 (2009).

[132] Flordal Thelander, E. et al. Detailed assessment of copy number alterations revealing homozygous deletions in 1p and 13q in mantle cell lymphoma. *Leukemia research* 31, 1219-1230, doi:10.1016/j.leukres.2006.10.022 (2007).

[133] Salaverria, I. et al. Specific secondary genetic alterations in mantle cell lymphoma provide prognostic information independent of the gene expression-based proliferation signature. *Journal of clinical oncology :*

*official journal of the American Society of Clinical Oncology* 25, 1216-1222, doi:10.1200/JCO.2006.08.4251 (2007).
[134] Kridel, R. et al. Whole transcriptome sequencing reveals recurrent NOTCH1 mutations in mantle cell lymphoma. *Blood* 119, 1963-1971, doi:10.1182/blood-2011-11-391474 (2012).
[135] Bea, S. et al. Landscape of somatic mutations and clonal evolution in mantle cell lymphoma. *Proceedings of the National Academy of Sciences of the United States of America* 110, 18250-18255, doi:10.1073/pnas.1314608110 (2013).
[136] Bernard, M. et al. Blastic variant of mantle cell lymphoma: a rare but highly aggressive subtype. *Leukemia* 15, 1785-1791 (2001).
[137] Salaverria, I., Perez-Galan, P., Colomer, D. & Campo, E. Mantle cell lymphoma: from pathology and molecular pathogenesis to new therapeutic perspectives. *Haematologica* 91, 11-16 (2006).
[138] Zelenetz, A. D. Mantle cell lymphoma: an update on management. *Annals of oncology : official journal of the European Society for Medical Oncology / ESMO* 17 Suppl 4, iv12-14, doi:10.1093/annonc/mdj992 (2006).
[139] Orchard, J. et al. A subset of t(11;14) lymphoma with mantle cell features displays mutated IgVH genes and includes patients with good prognosis, nonnodal disease. *Blood* 101, 4975-4981, doi:10.1182/blood-2002-06-1864 (2003).
[140] Argatoff, L. H., Connors, J. M., Klasa, R. J., Horsman, D. E. & Gascoyne, R. D. Mantle cell lymphoma: a clinicopathologic study of 80 cases. *Blood* 89, 2067-2078 (1997).
[141] Bosch, F. et al. Mantle cell lymphoma: presenting features, response to therapy, and prognostic factors. *Cancer* 82, 567-575 (1998).
[142] Katzenberger, T. et al. The Ki67 proliferation index is a quantitative indicator of clinical risk in mantle cell lymphoma. *Blood* 107, 3407, doi:10.1182/blood-2005-10-4079 (2006).
[143] Rosenwald, A. et al. The proliferation gene expression signature is a quantitative integrator of oncogenic events that predicts survival in mantle cell lymphoma. *Cancer cell* 3, 185-197 (2003).
[144] Martinez, N. et al. The molecular signature of mantle cell lymphoma reveals multiple signals favoring cell survival. *Cancer research* 63, 8226-8232 (2003).
[145] Vater, I. et al. GeneChip analyses point to novel pathogenetic mechanisms in mantle cell lymphoma. *British journal of haematology* 144, 317-331, doi:10.1111/j.1365-2141.2008.07443.x (2009).

[146] Cuneo, A. et al. Cytogenetic profile of lymphoma of follicle mantle lineage: correlation with clinicobiologic features. *Blood* 93, 1372-1380 (1999).

[147] Weisenburger, D. D. et al. Mantle cell lymphoma. A clinicopathologic study of 68 cases from the Nebraska Lymphoma Study Group. *American journal of hematology* 64, 190-196 (2000).

[148] Hoster, E. et al. A new prognostic index (MIPI) for patients with advanced-stage mantle cell lymphoma. *Blood* 111, 558-565, doi:10.1182/blood-2007-06-095331 (2008).

In: Mantle Cell Lymphoma
Editor: Charles L. Schmidt
ISBN: 978-1-63482-363-0


*Chapter 2*

# Mantle Cell Lymphoma: Current Treatment Strategies in the Era of Targeted Agents

***Muhammad Omer Jamil*[1*], *Maira Rizwan*[†], *and Amitkumar Mehta*[2‡]**
[1]Hematology & Oncology, Department of Medicine,
University of Alabama at Birmingham, Birmingham, AL, US
[2]Hematology & Oncology, Department of Medicine,
University of Alabama at Birmingham, Birmingham, AL, US

## Abstract

Mantle cell lymphoma (MCL) is a subtype of Non-Hodgkin's Lymphoma (NHL) with varying clinical presentations, ranging from indolent disease to highly aggressive clinical course. The MCL cells exhibit a characteristic translocation t(11;14) which juxtaposes immunoglobulin heavy chain gene with gene for cyclin D1 leading to overexpression of cyclin D1 which can be identified by

* Email:mjamil@uabmc.edu
† Email:dearestmeer@hotmail.com
‡ Corresponding Author: Email: amitkumarmehta@uabmc.edu; Phone: 205-996-8400, Fax: 205-934-1608.

immunohistochemistry and is useful as a diagnostic marker. Advancement in understanding of the biology and pathogenesis of MCL has led to discovery of multiple other genetic alterations impacting the cell cycle deregulation and development of sub clonal populations with certain genetic mutations (p53, ATM, NOTCH2) leading to disease progression and refractoriness to treatment. Mantle cell lymphoma international prognostic index (MIPI) and biologic MIPI (bMIPI) are prognostic indices to categorize indolent vs aggressive disease. Currently an intensive cytarabine containing upfront induction regimen followed with or without autologous transplant is recommended for younger and fit patients. Older or frail patients are thought to benefit more from less intensive rituximab containing regimens followed by rituximab maintenance. A small subset of patients with indolent disease can be observed. Most patients unfortunately relapse. Targeted molecular therapies (bortezomib, lenalidomide, ibrutinib, idelalsib etc.) have shown significant response rates in relapsed and refractory disease and are being evaluated further.

## Introduction

Mantle cell lymphoma (MCL) is a B cell Non Hodgkin Lymphoma (NHL) derived from CD5+ antigen naïve pregerminal center B cells within the mantle zone that surrounds the normal germinal center follicles. It comprises of about 6% of newly diagnosed NHL cases. [1] Median age at diagnoses is 68 years with male more commonly affected then females. [1, 2] The median survival is less than 5 years despite improvement in treatments and supportive care. [3] An excisional biopsy of involved lymph node or biopsy of the involved extra lymphatic site is required to make the diagnoses. [4] The hallmark of MCL is presence of t (11:14) which lead to upregulaiton of cyclin D1 (the first event in lymphomagenesis). [5] Certain cyclin D1 negative MCL can be diagnosed with the presence of SOX11, over expression of cyclin D2 and D3 which are not specific to MCL but may be helpful. [6-8]. It classically comprises of small to medium sized lymphocytes. Other histologic variants exist namely small cell variant, blastoid variant and pleomorphic variant. Immunophenotype of MCL is positive for B cell marker CD19, CD20, CD22 and CD79a, aberrant T cell markers CD5 and CD43 and negative for CD5. [9] MCL in situ has been defined with presence of MCL cells in mantle zone of reactive lymph node but the clinical significance of this entity is unclear at this time. [10] Although incurable with currently available approaches, newer targeted therapies are promising. In this chapter we will discuss factors impacting prognosis, targetable biologic pathways and treatment of MCL.

# Prognostic Indicators for MCL

Various different marker have been evaluated for MCL and been shown of importance. These include patient associated as well as tumor associated factors. The performance status of a patient at diagnosis is the most important factor as it determines the eligibility of patient to receive intensive vs less intensive chemotherapy. In one study patients with and eastern cooperative group performance score (ECOG PS) of equal to or more than 2 had a poor outcome. [11] Similar findings have been shown in a recent study which also revealed negative impact of male gender and B symptoms on survival. [12] Other factors like LDH, age at diagnosis and WBC count are also known to impact survival and thus are included in MCL International Prognostic Index (MIPI) (Figure 1). [13] It divides patients in low, intermediate and high risk group which are associated with 60%, 35% and 20% five year overall survival respectively. The mitotic rate of the lymphoma as measured by Ki67 expression has been shown to be directly related to survival. [14] and thus has been incorporated in biologic MIPI which incorporates Ki67 expression by adding one point for equal to or more than 30% Ki67 expression to MIPI score and exhibits similar predictive value. [13]

| Points | 0 | 1 | 2 | 3 |
|---|---|---|---|---|
| Age | <50 | 50-59 | 60-69 | ≥70 |
| ECOG | 0-1 | | 2-4 | |
| LDH (ULN) | <0.67 | 0.67-0.99 | 1-1.49 | ≥1.5 |
| WBC ($X10^9/L$) | <6.7 | 6.7-9.9 | 1-14.9 | ≥15 |

(* Modified & adapted from: Hoster E et al., Blood 2008. [13]).

Figure 1. Mantle cell lymphoma international prognostic index (MIPI).*

The cytologic characteristics of the lymphoma also have prognostic significance. The blastoid variant carries worse prognosis as compared to small cell variant. In a retrospective study 187 patients, 33 patients with blastoid variant had a worse overall survival at 14.5 months vs 53 months. [15] In another study, patients with the blastoid MCL subtype were more resistant to initial chemotherapy with response duration of 11 months vs 28 with a shorter overall survival (20 months vs. 42 months respectively). [16]

The blastoid variant is associated with higher Ki67 expression. [14, 17] Genetic alterations especially TP53 gene mutation or 17p13 deletion is also linked with worse outcomes in MCL patients. These abnormalities are more commonly seen in patients with blastoid variant of MCL. [18, 19].

# Cellular Pathways and Potential Targets for Therapy

The aggressive clinical behavior, rapid relapse and short response to treatment of MCL are related to multiple abnormalities found in cell cycle regulation, DNA damage repair, cell survival and apoptosis. [20] The proposed model of MCL lymphomagenesis and progression along with suggested treatment algorithm is depicted in Figure 2. Cyclin D1 (CCND1) translocation is the primary event followed by the activation of two major molecular signaling pathways namely INK4a/CDK4/RB1 and MDM2/p53/p27. This activation if likely further reinforced by other genetic alteration which lead to enhanced cell proliferation, resistance to apoptosis, immune evasion and interactions with tumor microenvironment via constitutive activation Wnt, hedgehog, PI3K/AKT/mammalian target of rapamycin (mTOR), B cell antigen receptor (BCR) and nuclear factor kappa-B (NF-κB) pathways as well as TP53 and BMI 1 amplification. [18] These pathways provide us with understanding of lymphomagenesis in MCL and also pose as potential targets of therapy. The overexpressed CCND1 complexes with CDK4 and CDK6, which leads to important downstream effect. The CCND1-CDK4 or CDK6 complex leads to phosphorylation of RB1 which in turn via the release of elongation factor 2(EF2) advances the cells into S phase. [5] The CCND1-CDK4 complex also inhibits the ability of CDK inhibitor p27 to cause G1 phase cell cycle arrest. [5]

The secondary genetic alterations are significant as they lead to more aggressive phenotype and resistance to chemotherapy. One of the secondary alterations is mutation of ataxia telangiectasia mutant gene (ATM), which is present in about 40% of MCL cases. ATM gene inactivation leads to impaired DNA damage response. Phosphatidyl inositol 3 Kinase (PI3K), which is a key kinase in this pathway is encoded by ATM gene as well. The PI3K-AKT pathway is notably located upstream from the mTOR pathway which in is turn upstream from the CCND1, p27 and other regulatory proteins. [21, 22]

Other pathways affected due to the genetic alteration include Wnt Canonical Pathway (WCP) via β-catenin and the hedgehog pathway. [23] The Sonic Hedgehog (SHH) is a known ligand for the hedgehog pathway and SHH-GLI molecules such as PTCH, SMO, GLI1 and GLI2 are expressed in MCL cell lines. Down regulation of GLI via inhibitory molecules have shown to decrease proliferation and increased susceptibility to chemotherapy in MCL. [24]

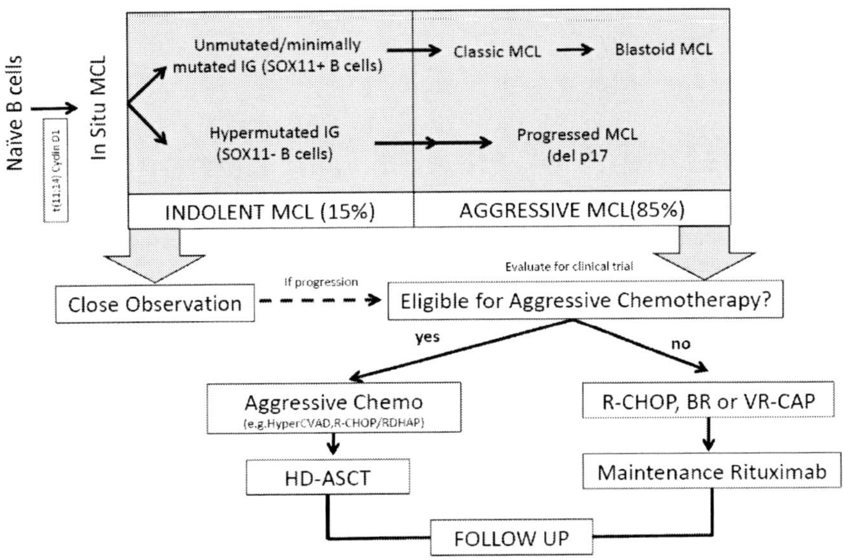


Abbreviations: R-CHOP:Rituximab, Cyclophosphamide, Doxorubicin, Prednisone, R-DHAP: Rituximab, Dexamethasone, Ara C, Carboplatin, ASCT: Autologus Stem Cell Transplant, R-HyperCVAD: Part A: Cyclophosphamide, Doxorubicin, Vincristine, Dexamethasone, Part B: Methotraxate, Ara C, BR: Bendamustine,Rituximab, VR-CAP: Bortezomib, Rituximab, Cyclophosphamide, Doxorubicin, Prednisone.

(Adapted from ASCO EdBook Mantle cell Lymphoma 2014; P Jares,Genetic and molecular pathogenesis of Mantle cell Lymphoma, 2007; P jares, Molecular pathogenesis of Mantle cell lymphoma, JCI, 2012).

Figure 2. MCL lymphomagenesis and treatment.

Ubiquitin proteasome pathway is a major non-lysosomal pathway via which cellular proteins are degraded. It plays critical role in cell cycle regulation via its effects on cyclins, CDKs and NF-κB. [25, 26] Persistent activity of NF-κB is due to tumor formation, tumor growth, metastasis and resistance to chemotherapy in different cancer type including B cell lymphomas. Inhibitors of this pathway has shown to have significant activity in treatment of MCL. [27, 28]

Recent studies have demonstrated the constitutive activation of BCR signal transduction in MCL. [29] Various studies have targeted BCR signal transduction with small molecule inhibitors of spleen tyrosine kinase (Syk), Brtuon's tyrosine kinase (Btk) and protein kinase C beta (PKC-β). Btk is a Tec family, non-receptor tyrosine kinase with a well-defined role in MCL development. Inhibitors of Btk are already proven to be efficacious in treatment of MCL. [30]

## Treatment of Mantle Cell Lymphoma

Mantle cell lymphoma is considered incurable with currently available treatment options. MCL has wide spectrum of clinical presentation ranging from indolent disease to symptomatic aggressive disease.

| Stage | Features |
|---|---|
| I | Involvement of a single lymph node region or lymphoid structure |
| II | Involvement of two or more lymph node regions or localized involvement of one extranodal site and one or lymph node regions (same side of diaphragm) |
| III | Involvement of lymph node regions or structures (both sides of the diaphragm) |
| IV | Diffuse or disseminated involvement of one or more extralymphatic organs/any involvement of the liver, bone marrow, pleura or CSF |

| Suffix | Description |
|---|---|
| A | Absence of constitutional symptoms |
| B | Constitutional symptoms: fever (> 38°C), drenching sweats, weight loss (10% body weight over 6 months) |
| E | Involvement of a single, extranodal site contiguous or proximal to a known nodal site |
| S | Splenic involvement |
| X | Bulky disease, defined as one or more site of disease of > 10 cm diameter, or mediastinal widening to > 1/3 of the chest width on chest X-ray |

Lister TA et al., JCO 1989. [35].

Figure 3. Ann Arbor staging of Non Hodgkin Lymphoma.

Indolent disease usually presents with limited stage disease, low tumor burden, without high risk features and low Ki67 expression. It has much better outcomes with prolonged overall survival. [6, 31-33]

Most patients will present with advanced disease and symptomatic disease thus will require treatment with intensive chemotherapy followed by consolidation. MCL also has tendency to involve gut mucosa in about 7-8% cases. [34] Ann Arbor staging system (updated with recent Lugano classification. [4] (Figure 3) is frequently used to stage MCL. [35]

# First Line therapy

## Limited Stage Disease (Ann Arbor Stage I-II)

Few patients present with localized MCL and there is not much literature available to help clinicians make decision for treatment. In one retrospective analysis (n=26), patients with limited stage (stage IA or IIA) nonbulky disease had improved progression free survival (PFS) at 5 years (68% vs 11%, P=0.002) and a trend towards improved overall survival (OS) when treated with radiation therapy with or without chemotherapy. [36] At this time in absence of more definitive data this patient group can be treated with radiation therapy alone or in combination with chemo immunotherapy.

## Extensive Disease (Stage II Bulky and Stage III-IV)

Treatment strategy for patients with extensive disease is based on multiple disease and patient related factor. Disease with high risk morphologic (e.g., blastoid variant) or genetic factors (e.g., del 17p) require more intensive therapy but this is not always the case as the median age of presentation of MCL is >65 years and patients often would have poor ECOG PS to tolerate intensive treatment.

Thus the choice of first line treatment is based mainly on the patient's ability to tolerate Aggressive chemotherapy.

## Aggressive First Line Therapy

Rituximab combined with high dose cytarabine followed by autologous hematopoietic transplantation (autoHSCT) is currently considered standard in treatment of MCL for fit patients. [37] The addition of rituximab to chemotherapy has been shown to be associated with improved response rates and PFS. [38] In a randomized controlled trial of CHOP vs R-CHOP, it was demonstrated that the addition of rituximab leads to better outcomes. [39] Other studies have also revealed similar results in terms of improvements in response rates, OS and PFS. [40] In patients with extensive blood involvement with MCL, the first dose of rituximab should be delivered with caution as it can be associated with cytokine storm or tumor lysis syndrome. Over the past decade multiple studies have revealed the role of cytarabine in treatment of MCL. Treatment regimens containing high dose cytarabine are shown to produce better complete response rates and PFS. [41-44] In a phase III trial comparing RCHOP(6 cycles) vs RCHOP(3 cycles) alternating with RDHAP(rituximab, dexamethasone, cytarabine and cisplatin)(3 cycles) followed by autologous transplantation, the patients in the alternating RCHOP/RDHAP showed better CR rate(25% vs 36%, p=0.012), longer response duration (46 vs. 48 months, $p$=0.0382) and longer overall survival (82 months vs. not reached, $p$=0.045). [45] In a phase II trial, R HyperCVAD (rituximab, cyclophosphamide, doxorubicin, vincristine and dexamethasone) alternating with R-MA (rituximab, methotrexate and cytarabine) was used to treat MCL in first line.

This regimen was associated with 97% response rate and CR rate of 87% and at 10 years follow up the median OS was not reached with median time to failure of 4.6 years. [46] A phase II study of trial of 49 patients treated for MCL in first line with R-HyperCVAD showed complete remission and unconfirmed complete remission rate was 58% with PFS and OS of 63% and 76% respectively. [47]

Another phase II Italian study has shown similar activity of this regimen. [48] Although highly active, R-HyperCVAD is associated with significant treatment related toxicity and interruption in therapy. Other intensive regimens like Nordic regimen, RCHOP/RICE and CALGB regimen have shown good results. [41, 49, 50] (table)

## Less Aggressive First Line Therapy

The standard of care at this time for patients with MCL who cannot tolerate aggressive first line treatment is chemo immunotherapy with regimens like RCHOP or BR (bendamustine and rituximab). A phase II international trial by European MCL network tested RCHOP against FCR (fludarabine, cyclophosphamide and rituximab) followed by second maintenance randomization between Interferon and rituximab [51]. The median overall survival at 4 years was significantly better in favor of the RCHOP arm (62% vs 47%, p=0.005). Higher number of deaths in the fludarabine arm were associated with disease relapse or infections. In second randomization, rituximab maintenance reduced risk of progression or death by 45 %( 68% vs 29%) and almost double the duration of response (in remission after 4 years, 58%, vs. 29% with interferon alfa; hazard ratio for progression or death, 0.55; 95% confidence interval, 0.36 to 0.87; P=0.01) and improved overall survival survival rates at 4 years were 79% in the rituximab group and 67% in the interferon alfa group (P=0.13). Favorable outcome have also been achieved with use of RCHOP followed by radio immunotherapy. [52]

Bendamustine in combination with rituximab have shown promising results in first line and relapse refractory setting. In a randomized phase III trial of BR vs RCHOP, BR showed significant improvement in PFS (35.4vs 22.1months) although there was no statistically significant difference in OS. [53] The combination of bendamustine and rituximab with cytarabine was evaluated in a Phase II study of patients older than 65 who were not eligible for aggressive chemotherapy. [54] Both previously untreated and patient who had received rituximab based regimen were included in the study, among untreated patients the ORR was 100% and the 2 year PFS was 95%. Among treated patients ORR was 70% with PFS of 70% at 2 years. A phase III double-blind study of ibrutinib in combination with BR versus BR for the treatment of patients with newly diagnosed MCL is currently ongoing (NCT01776840). [55]

Bortezomib, a proteasome inhibitor, inhibits 26S proteasome. By doing so, it inhibits NF-kB pathway making it rationale for activity in MCL. It was approved as a single agent, by US food and drug administration (US FDA) in MCL in relapse refractory setting in December 2006. In October, 2014, US FDA approved it in frontline setting in combination with rituximab, cyclophosphamide, doxorubicin and prednisone (VR-CAP). In the registration phase III trial, newly diagnosed MCL patients, not eligible for aggressive chemotherapy were randomized to receive VR-CAP or RCHOP. [56] At follow-up of 4 years VR-CAP patients had better PFS (24.7 vs 14.4 months, p=<0.001) and median OS (64% vs 54% for RCHOP at 4 years). Cladribine alone or in combination with rituximab has shown activity in untreated MCL. In a trial using single agent cladribine the overall response rate was 84 %( CR=42%) with a PFS of 14 months. [57] Other trials have shown similar results with single agent cladribine or combination with rituximab. [58, 59]

## First Line Consolidation Therapy

Intensive consolidation chemotherapy and high dose chemotherapy followed by autologous transplantation are usually not recommended for patients who above age 65 or who are unfit for such regimens. In much selected elderly patients however, this may be an acceptable option. [60] Autologous HSCT is now considered a standard consolidation strategy for young and fit patients with MCL. In a prospective study of frontline RCHOP/RDHAP followed by AutoHSCT the 3 year even free survival and overall survival were 84% and 90% respectively but the median overall survival not reached. [61] In this trial, the molecular reemission at 2 years post autoHSCT was associated with improvement in PFS and OS.

The only randomized trial evaluating myeloablative preconditioning chemo-radiotherapy followed by autoHSCT versus interferon-α (n=122), showed improvement in PFS (median 39 vs. 17 months, *p*=0.01) in favor of myeloablative chemo-radiotherapy but no difference in OS at 3 years (83 vs. 77%, *p*=0.18). [62] The MD Anderson group published a study of Hyper CVAD induction followed by consolidative autoHSCT which showed fiver year disease free survival of 42% and OS of 77%. Interestingly the patients with low Beta 2 microglobulin benefited the most by AutoHSCT in this study. [63] In the Nordic MCL-2 phase II trial, 160 MCL patients younger than 66 years were given 6 cycles of rituximab and high-dose cytarabine containing induction regimen followed by BEAM (carmustine, etoposide, cytarabine and melphalan) conditioning regimen and autoHSCT. The CR rate increased from 56% to 90% after myeloablative chemotherapy stressing the role of intensive consolidation therapy in improving the response rate. [41] In the European MCL Network phase III trial, the response rate after autoHSCT was 97% in the two arms but the rate of molecular remission that is a powerful and independent prognostic factor for the duration of the response rose from 55 to 72% after ASCT (*p*=0.0116). [45, 64]

The BEAM regimen is the commonly used conditioning regimen for autoHSCT mainly due to its convenience. Total body irradiation (TBI) is not recommended although some studies have shown its beneficial role in patients with partial response to induction chemotherapy. [65]

# Post Induction Maintenance Therapy

Maintenance therapy with rituximab may provide extended disease control in patients who are unable to undergo aggressive chemotherapy and/or autoHSCT. In a pilot phase II study, previously untreated patients with MCL were treated with modified less intense HyperCVAD followed but rituximab maintenance for 5 years. The median PFS was 37 months and median OS was not reached in favor of rituximab maintenance. [66] In another study of modified HyperCVAD with bortezomib followed by rituximab maintenance, median PFS and OS were not reached at 4 years. [67] The European lymphoma network trial evaluated rituximab vs interferon maintenance. It showed remarkable improvement in PFS and OS with RCHOP followed by rituximab maintenance. [68] This study suggests that patients who are not candidates for aggressive first line chemotherapy or autoHSCT, RCHOP followed by Rituximab maintenance is a reasonable option.

# Salvage Therapy for Relapsed or Refractory MCL

Relapsed or refractory MCL poses a daunting therapeutic challenge. The CR rates with available regimens are relatively low (<30%) with short responses. Various agents alone or in combinations have been tried for treatment of relapsed/refractory MCL. Bortezomib has been used with some success and is currently approved for treatment of relapsed MCL (US FDA approval December 2008). This approval was based on the PINNACLE trial, which was a phase II trial single agent bortezomib in treatment of relapsed/refractory MCL. It produced ORR of 33% with a median duration of response (MDR) of 9 months. [25] Median OS on long term follow up was 23.5 months in all patient and 35 months in patients who responded to treatment. [69] Smaller studies with bortezomib in combination with rituximab have also shown promising results. [70, 71]. Bendamustine alone or in combination with rituximab has shown activity in relapsed/refractory MCL. In a phase II multicenter trial of BR in treatment of relapsed refractory indolent or mantle cell lymphomas, ORR of 92% (42%CR) was observed in this heavily pretreated population. MDR was 19 months for MCL patients. [72] In a phase III randomized trial of BR vs FR (fludarabine and R) for treatment of patients with relapsed/refractory NHL including MCL, BR showed superior ORR of 83.5% (38.5%CR) and median PFS at 30 months. [73] Similar result shave been observed with combination of BR with bortezomib. [74] Lenalidomide is an immune modulating agent that has been evaluated in treatment of relapsed/refractory aggressive NHL. In subset analysis of a phase II trial (NHL-002) of single agent lenalidomide, the ORR was 53 %( 20%CR) with MDR and PFS of 14 and 6 months respectively. [75] Similar findings were observed in analysis of a larger NHL-003 study. [76, 77] A dedicated phase II study to evaluate lenalidomide in treatment of relapsed refractory MCL showed ORR of 31% with MRD of 20 months. [78] Lenalidomide has also been combined to rituximab, dexamethasone or bortezomib in phases I/II studies completing an ORR between 40 and 82% and MRD of about 18 months. [79-82] Ibrutinib is a small molecule inhibitor of Bruton's Tyrosine Kinase (BTK). BTK is a part of the B cell antigen receptor complex. It was evaluated in a phase I dose escalation trial in relapsed or refractory B cell malignancies. [83] In MCL subgroup, response was seen in 7 out of patients with 3 achieving CR with manageable toxicities. A recent phase II of ibrutinib in heavily pretreated MCL patients (n=111) showed ORR of 68% (21% CR). The median PFS was 8 months and median OS not reached. MDR was 17.5 months. [30] Ibrutinib affects homing leading to lymphocytosis in these patients which resolve in about 8 weeks. [84] Based on these findings US FDA granted Ibrutinib, a breakthrough therapy for MCL and eventually approved in this setting in November 2013.

## Second Line Consolidation Therapy

Consolidation with autoHSCT could be an option for patients who did not receive autoHSCT consolidation in the first line and are eligible for HSCT. However, the outcome of patients remains poor with a median duration of response around 2 years. [85] In a retrospective study of 195 patients from the European Blood and Marrow Transplantation (EBMT) registry and Autologous Blood and Marrow Transplant Registry (ABMTR), data was collected for patients who received autologous HSCT for MCL from year

1988-1998,a 5-year PFS and OS of 33% and 50% respectively was demonstrated. [86] The incorporation of radioimmunotherapy into the conditioning regimen has improved ORR, MRD and PFS. [87, 88]. For young and fit post autoHSCT relapse, with available HLA-identical donor, reduced intensity (RIC) allogeneic bone marrow transplant (alloHSCT) is an option with a potential of cure and acceptable transplant-related mortality (TRM). [38, 89]

In two large trials, the TRM at 2 and 5 years was 24 and 21% respectively and the PFS and OS at 2 and 5 years were 60 and 14% and 65 and 37% respectively. [58, 90] A retrospective study from the ESBMT registry of 279 patients who underwent RIC alloHSCT between 1998 and 2007 showed a 1 and 3 year PFS of 49% and 29% respectively and OS of 6°% and 43% respectively. [91] More recently, another survey from the ESBMT registry evaluated the outcome of patients (n=360, 80 with allo HSCT) with MCL relapsing after autoHSCT. With a median observation of 32 months, the 2 and 5-year survival was 46% and 34% respectively compared to 37% and 16% for patients without alloHSCT. [92] Based on these studies, alloHSCT is a potential option for transplant eligible patients.

## Novel Agents in Treatment of MCL

With advent of our understanding of the pathobiology of MCL and the cellular pathways linked to its aggressive behavior and resistance of conventional chemotherapeutic agents newer targets are recognized and novel agents are being developed.

### Bruton's Tyrosine Kinase (BTK) Inhibition

BTK is one of the downstream mediator of BCR function. BTK play a critical role in signal transduction which leads to tumor growth and proliferation. [93] Ibrutinib is a potent inhibitor of BTK. It has shown to have clinically significant activity in treatment of relapse/refractory MCL. [30, 83] and is currently approved for this indication. It is now being investigated in frontline setting in MCL treatment.

## Spleen Tyrosine Kinase (SYK) Inhibition

SYK is a part of the BCR complex. It leads to downstream activation of BTK. Rinaldi et al., have shown that MCL lymphocytes have overexpression of SYK due to increased transcription of the gene. [94] SYK inhibitors are currently available for use in clinical trial and are being tested in treatment of B cell NHL. Fostamatinib, a SYK inhibitor, has shown modest activity as single agent in relapsed refractory MCL (ORR of 11%). [95]

## PI3Kδ Inhibition

Two class I PI3K isoforms inhibitors have been tested for relapsed MCL, the oral isoform-selective inhibitor PI3K (CAL-101/ GS-1101, idelalisib) that blocks survival signals, induces apoptosis and disrupts signals between the tumor microenvironment and B-cell malignancies. [96-98] and the more pleiotropic PI3K- (Copanlisib/BAY 80 – 6946) that exhibits preferential inhibition of AKT phosphorylation, superior antitumor activity and potent apoptosis inducing activity. [99]

A phase I trial of Idelalisib, in heavily pretreated patients with MCL confirmed the activity of this compound with an ORR of 40% (5% CR) and a 1-year PFS of 22%. [100] Copanlisib, an intravenous formulations has been evaluated in a phase II study in various lymphomas, including 7 patients with MCL with ORR of 71% (1 uCR / 4 PR). [101]

## Mammalian Target of Rapamycin (mTOR) Inhibition

Temsirolimus is an mTOR inhibitor with antiproliferative and antioangiogenic effects that blocks the PI3K signaling pathway resulting in the cell cycle arrest and apoptosis. [102] Based on encouraging phase II trials demonstrating the efficacy of temsirolimus in the treatment of MCL patients [103, 104], a phase III trial was formulated comparing temsirolimus in two differenst dosing schedule vs investigator's choice of chemotherapy. Temsirolimus was randomly given at one of two different schedules (175 mg weekly for 3 weeks followed by either 75 mg or 25 mg weekly) and compared to investigator's choice monotherapy (gemcitabine (42%) or fludarabine (27%)). The 175/75 mg group was associated with the best response rate (22 vs. 2%) and a prolonged OS (12, 8 vs. 9, 7 months) over the investigator's choice group. [105] Based on this results, Temsirolimus is approved in Europe by EMA. Temsirolimus has also been investigated in combination with other drugs. In a phase II study reported by Ansell and colleagues, 69 patients with relapsed or refractory MCL were treated with Rituximab (375 mg/m$^2$/week) and temsirolimus (25 mg/week). The ORR was 59% (CR=19%). [106]

## BCL2 Inhibitor

BCl2 is known to be up regulated in patients with MCL and leads o increased cell survival and resistance to apoptosis. ABT-199 is an orally bioavailable, second-generation BCL2-specific BH3 mimetic that has demonstrated antitumor activity in a phase I study of 31 patients with NHL. All eight patients with MCL ạchieved PR. [107] A phase 1b multicenter study of ABT-199 in combination with BR in patients with relapsed/refractory NHL is underway.

## New Monoclonal Antibodies (mAB)

The first glycolengineered type II antibody, obinutuzumab (GA101), induces cell death and antibody-dependent cellular cytotoxicity in a different manner than type I antibodies (rituximab and ofatumumab). [108] A recent phase II GAUGUIN study of two doses of obinutuzumab monotherapy in relapsed/refractory diffuse large B-cell lymphoma and MCL reported response in 4 of 15 heavily pretreated MCL patients.

The most common adverse events were infusion-related reactions. [109] Ofatumumab, a fully humanized mAb that targets a unique epitope on the CD20 and has superior complement-dependent cytotoxicity compared with rituximab. [110-112] Preliminary results from a multicenter phase I/II study of ofatumumab plus bendamustine and dexamethasone in newly diagnosed older MCL patients showed ORR of 94% (CR :90%) in 19 evaluable patients with very high molecular CR. [110]

| | Regimen | Phase | No. Of Patients | ORR%(CR%) | PFS | OS |
|---|---|---|---|---|---|---|
| Intense therapy for eligible patients | CHOP±R f/b ASCT vs Interferonα[62] | III | 122 | 98(81) vs 99(37) | 3.3 yrs vs 1.4yrs | NR (83% at 3 yrs) vs NR (77% 3 yrs) |
| | RCHOP f/b ASCT vs RCHOP/RDHAP f/b ASCT[118] | III | 455 | 98(63) vs 97(61) | 3.8 yrs vs 7.3 yrs | 6.8 vs NR |
| | R-Hyper CVAD[119] | II | 97 | 97(87) | 4.6 yrs | NR (46% at 10 yrs) |
| | R-HyperCVAD[48] | II | 60 | 83(72) | NR (73% at 5 yrs) | NR (61% at 5 yrs) |
| Less intense therapy | BR Vs R-CHOP,R-CVP[120] | III (NI) | 447 (MCL,n=74) | 71%(for iNHL and MCL), CR ratio 1.95 (in favor of BR-40%, p=0.017) | NR | NR |
| | BR vs R-CHOP[121] | III | 549 | 93 (40) vs 91(30) for all patients | 35.4 mths vs 22.1 mths | No difference |
| | VR-CAP vs R-CHOP[56] | III | 487 | (42%vs 28%) | 30.7mths vs 16.7mths at 4 yrs | 64% at 4 yrs vs 54% at 4yrs |
| Mainten-ance | R-CHOP vs R-FC f/b R maintenance vs Interferonα[51] | III | 485 | 86(34) vs 78(40) | 28 mths vs 26 mths (TTF) | 62 vs 47 (at 4 yrs) |
| | | R maintenance vs Interferonα | | | | 79 vs 67 (at 4 yrs) |

Abbreviations: R-CHOP:Rituximab, Cyclophosphamide, Doxorubicin, Prednisone, R-DHAP: Rituximab, Dexamethasone, Ara C, Carboplatin, ASCT: Autologus Stem Cell Transplant, R-HyperCVAD: Part A: Cyclophosphamide, Doxorubicin, Vincristine, Dexamethasone, Part B: Methotraxate, Ara C, R-CVP: Rituximab, Cyclophosphamide, Vincristine and Prednisone, R-FC: Rituximab, Fludarabine and Cyclophosphamide, f/b=followed by, NR: Not Reached, NI: Non Inferiority, mths: months, yrs: years, ORR: Overall Response rate, CR: Complete Response, PFS: Progression Free Survival, OS: Overall Survival, TTF: Time to treatment failure, MCL: Mantle cell Lymphoma, iNHL (indolent non Hodgkin lymphoma).

Figure 4. Summary of recommended treatments for MCL.

### Other Novel Agents and Combination

Other promising agents in early-phase trials include: the CDK4/6 inhibitor PD0332991 [113], the histone deacetylase inhibitors (vorinostat [114] and abexinostat [115]) the farnesyltransferase inhibitor (tipifarnib [116]), and the anti-CD79 conjugated mAb DCDS4501A117.

## Conclusion

In summary, the treatment of MCL is in rapid evolution phase. Patients with limited disease should be treated with radiation therapy with or without chemotherapy. Fit-patients with advanced disease should undergo aggressive first line treatment followed by consolidative autoHSCT. For unfit-patients, RCHOP, BR or VR-CAP followed by maintenance therapy with rituximab is the best option.

Various different regimens are available for relapsed/refractory MCL. With more promising agents in clinical trials, enrolling the patient in a protocol is the best option. For fit-patients with relapse/refractory MCL and with available donor, RIC alloHSCT is a reasonable choice. Increasing understanding of the underlying pathobiology of MCL has led to evolution of new targeted agents which offer much promise in the treatment of MCL. Future trials will help us to better risk stratify the individual patient, evaluate the role of HSCT, and incorporate the novel targeted therapeutic agents in the treatment of MCL.

## References

[1] A clinical evaluation of the International Lymphoma Study Group classification of non-Hodgkin's lymphoma. The Non-Hodgkin's Lymphoma Classification Project. *Blood*. 1997;89(11):3909-3918.

[2] Zhou Y, Wang H, Fang W, et al. Incidence trends of mantle cell lymphoma in the United States between 1992 and 2004. *Cancer*. 2008;113(4):791-798.

[3] Caballero D, Campo E, Lopez-Guillermo A, et al. Clinical practice guidelines for diagnosis, treatment, and follow-up of patients with

mantle cell lymphoma. Recommendations from the GEL/TAMO Spanish Cooperative Group. *Ann Hematol.* 2013;92(9):1151-1179.

[4] Cheson BD, Fisher RI, Barrington SF, Cavalli F, Schwartz LH, Lister TA. Recommendations for initial evaluation, staging, and response assessment of Hodgkin and non-Hodgkin lymphoma: the Lugano classification. *J Clin Oncol.* 2014;32(27):3059-3068.

[5] Jares P, Colomer D, Campo E. Molecular pathogenesis of mantle cell lymphoma. *J Clin Invest.* 2012;122(10):3416-3423.

[6] Mozos A, Royo C, Hartmann E, et al. SOX11 expression is highly specific for mantle cell lymphoma and identifies the cyclin D1-negative subtype. *Haematologica.* 2009;94(11):1555-1562.

[7] Wlodarska I, Dierickx D, Vanhentenrijk V, et al. Translocations targeting CCND2, CCND3, and MYCN do occur in t(11;14)-negative mantle cell lymphomas. *Blood.* 2008;111(12):5683-5690.

[8] Salaverria I, Royo C, Carvajal-Cuenca A, et al. CCND2 rearrangements are the most frequent genetic events in cyclin D1(-) mantle cell lymphoma. *Blood.* 2013;121(8):1394-1402.

[9] Weisenburger DD, Armitage JO. Mantle cell lymphoma-- an entity comes of age. *Blood.* 1996;87(11):4483-4494.

[10] Carvajal-Cuenca A, Sua LF, Silva NM, et al. In situ mantle cell lymphoma: clinical implications of an incidental finding with indolent clinical behavior. *Haematologica.* 2012;97(2):270-278.

[11] Bosch F, Lopez-Guillermo A, Campo E, et al. Mantle cell lymphoma: presenting features, response to therapy, and prognostic factors. *Cancer.* 1998;82(3):567-575.

[12] van de Schans SA, Janssen-Heijnen ML, Nijziel MR, Steyerberg EW, van Spronsen DJ. Validation, revision and extension of the Mantle Cell Lymphoma International Prognostic Index in a population-based setting. *Haematologica.* 2010;95(9):1503-1509.

[13] Hoster E, Dreyling M, Klapper W, et al. A new prognostic index (MIPI) for patients with advanced-stage mantle cell lymphoma. *Blood.* 2008;111(2):558-565.

[14] Raty R, Franssila K, Joensuu H, Teerenhovi L, Elonen E. Ki-67 expression level, histological subtype, and the International Prognostic Index as outcome predictors in mantle cell lymphoma. *Eur J Haematol.* 2002;69(1):11-20.

[15] Bernard M, Gressin R, Lefrere F, et al. Blastic variant of mantle cell lymphoma: a rare but highly aggressive subtype. *Leukemia.* 2001;15(11):1785-1791.

[16] Parrens M, Belaud-Rotureau MA, Fitoussi O, et al. Blastoid and common variants of mantle cell lymphoma exhibit distinct immunophenotypic and interphase FISH features. *Histopathology.* 2006;48(4):353-362.

[17] Klapper W, Hoster E, Determann O, et al. Ki-67 as a prognostic marker in mantle cell lymphoma-consensus guidelines of the pathology panel of the European MCL Network. *J Hematop.* 2009;2(2):103-111.

[18] Stefancikova L, Moulis M, Fabian P, et al. Loss of the p53 tumor suppressor activity is associated with negative prognosis of mantle cell lymphoma. *Int J Oncol.* 2010;36(3):699-706.

[19] Kienle D, Katzenberger T, Ott G, et al. Quantitative gene expression deregulation in mantle-cell lymphoma: correlation with clinical and biologic factors. *J Clin Oncol.* 2007;25(19):2770-2777.

[20] Perez-Galan P, Dreyling M, Wiestner A. Mantle cell lymphoma: biology, pathogenesis, and the molecular basis of treatment in the genomic era. *Blood.* 2011;117(1):26-38.

[21] Cecconi D, Zamo A, Bianchi E, et al. Signal transduction pathways of mantle cell lymphoma: a phosphoproteome-based study. *Proteomics.* 2008;8(21):4495-4506.

[22] Dal Col J, Zancai P, Terrin L, et al. Distinct functional significance of Akt and mTOR constitutive activation in mantle cell lymphoma. *Blood.* 2008;111(10):5142-5151.

[23] Gelebart P, Anand M, Armanious H, et al. Constitutive activation of the Wnt canonical pathway in mantle cell lymphoma. *Blood.* 2008;112(13):5171-5179.

[24] Hegde GV, Munger CM, Emanuel K, et al. Targeting of sonic hedgehog-GLI signaling: a potential strategy to improve therapy for mantle cell lymphoma. *Mol Cancer Ther.* 2008;7(6):1450-1460.

[25] Ishii Y, Waxman S, Germain D. Targeting the ubiquitin-proteasome pathway in cancer therapy. *Anticancer Agents Med Chem.* 2007;7(3):359-365.

[26] Palombella VJ, Rando OJ, Goldberg AL, Maniatis T. The ubiquitin-proteasome pathway is required for processing the NF-kappa B1 precursor protein and the activation of NF-kappa B. *Cell.* 1994;78(5):773-785.

[27] Fisher RI, Bernstein SH, Kahl BS, et al. Multicenter phase II study of bortezomib in patients with relapsed or refractory mantle cell lymphoma. *J Clin Oncol.* 2006;24(30):4867-4874.

[28] Kuhn DJ, Orlowski RZ, Bjorklund CC. Second generation proteasome inhibitors: carfilzomib and immunoproteasome-specific inhibitors (IPSIs). *Curr Cancer Drug Targets*. 2011;11(3):285-295.

[29] Refaeli Y, Young RM, Turner BC, Duda J, Field KA, Bishop JM. The B cell antigen receptor and overexpression of MYC can cooperate in the genesis of B cell lymphomas. *PLoS Biol*. 2008;6(6):e152.

[30] Wang ML, Rule S, Martin P, et al. Targeting BTK with ibrutinib in relapsed or refractory mantle-cell lymphoma. *N Engl J Med*. 2013;369(6):507-516.

[31] Tiemann M, Schrader C, Klapper W, et al. Histopathology, cell proliferation indices and clinical outcome in 304 patients with mantle cell lymphoma (MCL): a clinicopathological study from the European MCL Network. *Br J Haematol*. 2005;131(1):29-38.

[32] Angelopoulou MK, Siakantariz MP, Vassilakopoulos TP, et al. The splenic form of mantle cell lymphoma. *Eur J Haematol*. 2002;68(1):12-21.

[33] Martin P, Chadburn A, Christos P, et al. Outcome of deferred initial therapy in mantle-cell lymphoma. *J Clin Oncol*. 2009;27(8):1209-1213.

[34] Morton LM, Sampson JN, Cerhan JR, et al. Rationale and Design of the International Lymphoma Epidemiology Consortium (InterLymph) Non-Hodgkin Lymphoma Subtypes Project. *J Natl Cancer Inst Monogr*. 2014;2014(48):1-14.

[35] Lister TA, Crowther D, Sutcliffe SB, et al. Report of a committee convened to discuss the evaluation and staging of patients with Hodgkin's disease: Cotswolds meeting. *J Clin Oncol*. 1989;7(11):1630-1636.

[36] Leitch HA, Gascoyne RD, Chhanabhai M, Voss NJ, Klasa R, Connors JM. Limited-stage mantle-cell lymphoma. *Ann Oncol*. 2003;14(10):1555-1561.

[37] Dreyling M, Thieblemont C, Gallamini A, et al. ESMO Consensus conferences: guidelines on malignant lymphoma. part 2: marginal zone lymphoma, mantle cell lymphoma, peripheral T-cell lymphoma. *Ann Oncol*. 2013;24(4):857-877.

[38] Tam CS, Bassett R, Ledesma C, et al. Mature results of the M. D. Anderson Cancer Center risk-adapted transplantation strategy in mantle cell lymphoma. *Blood*. 2009;113(18):4144-4152.

[39] Lenz G, Dreyling M, Hoster E, et al. Immunochemotherapy with rituximab and cyclophosphamide, doxorubicin, vincristine, and prednisone significantly improves response and time to treatment failure,

but not long-term outcome in patients with previously untreated mantle cell lymphoma: results of a prospective randomized trial of the German Low Grade Lymphoma Study Group (GLSG). *J Clin Oncol.* 2005;23(9):1984-1992.

[40] Schulz H, Bohlius J, Skoetz N, et al. Chemotherapy plus Rituximab versus chemotherapy alone for B-cell non-Hodgkin's lymphoma. *Cochrane Database Syst Rev.* 2007(4):Cd003805.

[41] Geisler CH, Kolstad A, Laurell A, et al. Long-term progression-free survival of mantle cell lymphoma after intensive front-line immunochemotherapy with in vivo-purged stem cell rescue: a nonrandomized phase 2 multicenter study by the Nordic Lymphoma Group. *Blood.* 2008;112(7):2687-2693.

[42] Lefrere F, Delmer A, Levy V, Delarue R, Varet B, Hermine O. Sequential chemotherapy regimens followed by high-dose therapy with stem cell transplantation in mantle cell lymphoma: an update of a prospective study. *Haematologica.* 2004;89(10):1275-1276.

[43] Harel S, Delarue R, Ribrag V, Dreyling M, Hermine O. Treatment of younger patients with mantle cell lymphoma. *Semin Hematol.* 2011;48(3):194-207.

[44] Delarue R, Haioun C, Ribrag V, et al. CHOP and DHAP plus rituximab followed by autologous stem cell transplantation in mantle cell lymphoma: a phase 2 study from the Groupe d'Etude des Lymphomes de l'Adulte. *Blood.* 2013;121(1):48-53.

[45] Hermine O, Hoster E, Walewski J, et al. Alternating Courses of 3x CHOP and 3x DHAP Plus Rituximab Followed by a High Dose ARA-C Containing Myeloablative Regimen and Autologous Stem Cell Transplantation (ASCT) Increases Overall Survival When Compared to 6 Courses of CHOP Plus Rituximab Followed by Myeloablative Radiochemotherapy and ASCT in Mantle Cell Lymphoma: Final Analysis of the MCL Younger Trial of the European Mantle Cell Lymphoma Network (MCL net). 2012.

[46] Romaguera JE, Fayad LE, Feng L, et al. Ten-year follow-up after intense chemoimmunotherapy with Rituximab-HyperCVAD alternating with Rituximab-high dose methotrexate/cytarabine (R-MA) and without stem cell transplantation in patients with untreated aggressive mantle cell lymphoma. *Br J Haematol.* 2010;150(2):200-208.

[47] Bernstein SH, Epner E, Unger JM, et al. A phase II multicenter trial of hyperCVAD MTX/Ara-C and rituximab in patients with previously

untreated mantle cell lymphoma; SWOG 0213. *Ann Oncol.* 2013;24(6):1587-1593.

[48] Merli F, Luminari S, Ilariucci F, et al. Rituximab plus HyperCVAD alternating with high dose cytarabine and methotrexate for the initial treatment of patients with mantle cell lymphoma, a multicentre trial from Gruppo Italiano Studio Linfomi. *Br J Haematol.* 2012;156(3):346-353.

[49] Damon LE, Johnson JL, Niedzwiecki D, et al. Immunochemotherapy and autologous stem-cell transplantation for untreated patients with mantle-cell lymphoma: CALGB 59909. *J Clin Oncol.* 2009;27(36): 6101-6108.

[50] Schaffel R, Hedvat CV, Teruya-Feldstein J, et al. Prognostic impact of proliferative index determined by quantitative image analysis and the International Prognostic Index in patients with mantle cell lymphoma. *Ann Oncol.* 2010;21(1):133-139.

[51] Kluin-Nelemans HC, Hoster E, Hermine O, et al. Treatment of older patients with mantle-cell lymphoma. *N Engl J Med.* 2012;367(6):520-531.

[52] Smith MR, Li H, Gordon L, et al. Phase II study of rituximab plus cyclophosphamide, doxorubicin, vincristine, and prednisone immunochemotherapy followed by yttrium-90-ibritumomab tiuxetan in untreated mantle-cell lymphoma: Eastern Cooperative Oncology Group Study E1499. *J Clin Oncol.* 2012;30(25):3119-3126.

[53] Rummel MJ, Niederle N, Maschmeyer G, et al. Bendamustine plus rituximab versus CHOP plus rituximab as first-line treatment for patients with indolent and mantle-cell lymphomas: an open-label, multicentre, randomised, phase 3 non-inferiority trial. *Lancet.* 2013;381(9873):1203-1210.

[54] Visco C, Finotto S, Zambello R, et al. Combination of rituximab, bendamustine, and cytarabine for patients with mantle-cell non-Hodgkin lymphoma ineligible for intensive regimens or autologous transplantation. *J Clin Oncol.* 2013;31(11):1442-1449.

[55] Michael Wang LIG, Simon Rule, Andre Goy, Olivier Hermine, Aleksandra Rizo, Sen Hong Zhuang, Martin H. Dreyling. A phase III study of ibrutinib in combination with bendamustine and rituximab (BR) in elderly patients with newly diagnosed mantle cell lymphoma (MCL). *Journal of Clinical Oncology*. 2013.

[56] Franco Cavalli BR, Lixia Pei, Helgi Van De Velde, Tadeusz Robak,. Randomized phase 3 study of rituximab, cyclophosphamide, doxorubicin, and prednisone plus vincristine (R-CHOP) or bortezomib

(VR-CAP) in newly diagnosed mantle cell lymphoma (MCL) patients (pts) ineligible for bone marrow transplantation (BMT). *Journal of clinical oncology*. 2014;32(5):8500.

[57] Inwards DJ, Fishkin PA, Hillman DW, et al. Long-term results of the treatment of patients with mantle cell lymphoma with cladribine (2-CDA) alone (95-80-53) or 2-CDA and rituximab (N0189) in the North Central Cancer Treatment Group. *Cancer*. 2008;113(1):108-116.

[58] Rummel MJ, Chow KU, Jager E, et al. Treatment of mantle-cell lymphomas with intermittent two-hour infusion of cladribine as first-line therapy or in first relapse. *Ann Oncol*. 1999;10(1):115-117.

[59] Spurgeon SE, Pindyck T, Okada C, et al. Cladribine plus rituximab is an effective therapy for newly diagnosed mantle cell lymphoma. *Leuk Lymphoma*. 2011;52(8):1488-1494.

[60] Jantunen E, Canals C, Attal M, et al. Autologous stem-cell transplantation in patients with mantle cell lymphoma beyond 65 years of age: a study from the European Group for Blood and Marrow Transplantation (EBMT). *Ann Oncol*. 2012;23(1):166-171.

[61] Lefrere F, Delmer A, Suzan F, et al. Sequential chemotherapy by CHOP and DHAP regimens followed by high-dose therapy with stem cell transplantation induces a high rate of complete response and improves event-free survival in mantle cell lymphoma: a prospective study. *Leukemia*. 2002;16(4):587-593.

[62] Dreyling M, Lenz G, Hoster E, et al. Early consolidation by myeloablative radiochemotherapy followed by autologous stem cell transplantation in first remission significantly prolongs progression-free survival in mantle-cell lymphoma: results of a prospective randomized trial of the European MCL Network. *Blood*. 2005;105(7):2677-2684.

[63] Khouri IF, Saliba RM, Okoroji GJ, Acholonu SA, Champlin RE. Long-term follow-up of autologous stem cell transplantation in patients with diffuse mantle cell lymphoma in first disease remission: the prognostic value of beta2-microglobulin and the tumor score. *Cancer*. 2003; 98(12):2630-2635.

[64] Pott C, Hoster E, Delfau-Larue MH, et al. Molecular remission is an independent predictor of clinical outcome in patients with mantle cell lymphoma after combined immunochemotherapy: a European MCL intergroup study. *Blood*. 2010;115(16):3215-3223.

[65] Rubio MT, Boumendil A, Luan JJ, et al. Is There Still a Place for Total Body Irradiation (TBI) In the Conditioning Regimen of Autologous

Stem Cell Transplantation In Mantle Cell Lymphoma ?: a Retrospective Study From the Lymphoma Working Party of the EBMT. 2010.

[66] Kahl BS, Longo WL, Eickhoff JC, et al. Maintenance rituximab following induction chemoimmunotherapy may prolong progression-free survival in mantle cell lymphoma: a pilot study from the Wisconsin Oncology Network. *Ann Oncol.* 2006;17(9):1418-1423.

[67] Chang JE, Peterson C, Choi S, et al. VcR-CVAD induction chemotherapy followed by maintenance rituximab in mantle cell lymphoma: a Wisconsin Oncology Network study. *Br J Haematol.* 2011;155(2):190-197.

[68] !!! INVALID CITATION !!!

[69] Goy A, Bernstein SH, Kahl BS, et al. Bortezomib in patients with relapsed or refractory mantle cell lymphoma: updated time-to-event analyses of the multicenter phase 2 PINNACLE study. *Ann Oncol.* 2009;20(3):520-525.

[70] Baiocchi RA, Alinari L, Lustberg ME, et al. Phase 2 trial of rituximab and bortezomib in patients with relapsed or refractory mantle cell and follicular lymphoma. *Cancer.* 2011;117(11):2442-2451.

[71] Lamm W, Kaufmann H, Raderer M, et al. Bortezomib combined with rituximab and dexamethasone is an active regimen for patients with relapsed and chemotherapy-refractory mantle cell lymphoma. *Haematologica.* 2011;96(7):1008-1014.

[72] Robinson KS, Williams ME, van der Jagt RH, et al. Phase II multicenter study of bendamustine plus rituximab in patients with relapsed indolent B-cell and mantle cell non-Hodgkin's lymphoma. *J Clin Oncol.* 2008;26(27):4473-4479.

[73] Rummel MJ, Kaiser U, Balser C, et al. Bendamustine Plus Rituximab Versus Fludarabine Plus Rituximab In Patients with Relapsed Follicular, Indolent and Mantle Cell Lymphomas - Final Results of the Randomized Phase III Study NHL 2-2003 on Behalf of the StiL (Study Group Indolent Lymphomas, Germany). 2010.

[74] Friedberg JW, Vose JM, Kelly JL, et al. The combination of bendamustine, bortezomib, and rituximab for patients with relapsed/refractory indolent and mantle cell non-Hodgkin lymphoma. *Blood.* 2011;117(10):2807-2812.

[75] Habermann TM, Lossos IS, Justice G, et al. Lenalidomide oral monotherapy produces a high response rate in patients with relapsed or refractory mantle cell lymphoma. *Br J Haematol.* 2009;145(3):344-349.

[76] Reeder CB, Witzig TE, Zinzani PL, et al. Efficacy and safety of lenalidomide oral monotherapy in patients with relapsed or refractory mantle-cell lymphoma: Results from an international study (NHL-003). 2009.

[77] Zinzani PL, Vose JM, Czuczman MS, et al. Phase II Multicenter Study of the Safety and Efficacy of Single-Agent Lenalidomide in Subjects with Relapsed/Refractory Mantle Cell Lymphoma: Long-Term Follow-up Analysis of the NHL-003 Study. 2012.

[78] Eve HE, Carey S, Richardson SJ, et al. Single-agent lenalidomide in relapsed/refractory mantle cell lymphoma: results from a UK phase II study suggest activity and possible gender differences. *Br J Haematol.* 2012;159(2):154-163.

[79] Zaja F, De Luca S, Vitolo U, et al. Salvage treatment with lenalidomide and dexamethasone in relapsed/refractory mantle cell lymphoma: clinical results and effects on microenvironment and neo-angiogenic biomarkers. *Haematologica.* 2012;97(3):416-422.

[80] Wang M, Fayad L, Wagner-Bartak N, et al. Lenalidomide in combination with rituximab for patients with relapsed or refractory mantle-cell lymphoma: a phase 1/2 clinical trial. *Lancet Oncol.* 2012;13(7):716-723.

[81] Morrison VA, Jung S-H, Johnson J, et al. Salvage Therapy with Bortezomib Plus Lenalidomide for Relapsed/Refractory Mantle Cell Lymphoma: Initial Results of a Phase II Trial (Alliance/CALGB 50501). 2012.

[82] Flinn IW, Mainwaring M, Peacock N, et al. Rituximab, Lenalidomide, and Bortezomib in the First-Line or Second-Line Treatment of Patients with Mantle Cell Lymphoma a Phase I/II Trial. 2012.

[83] Advani RH, Buggy JJ, Sharman JP, et al. Bruton tyrosine kinase inhibitor ibrutinib (PCI-32765) has significant activity in patients with relapsed/refractory B-cell malignancies. *J Clin Oncol.* 2013;31(1):88-94.

[84] Ibrutinib prescription information. http://accessdta.fda.gov/drugsatfda_docs/label/2013/ 205552lbl.pdf.

[85] Swerdlow SH CE, Harris NL, et al. World Health Organization classification of tumors of haematopoietic and lymphoid tissues. Lyon: France IARC Press; 2008.

[86] Vandenberghe E, Ruiz de Elvira C, Loberiza FR, et al. Outcome of autologous transplantation for mantle cell lymphoma: a study by the European Blood and Bone Marrow Transplant and Autologous Blood

and Marrow Transplant Registries. *Br J Haematol.* 2003;120(5):793-800.

[87] Krishnan A, Nademanee A, Fung HC, et al. Phase II trial of a transplantation regimen of yttrium-90 ibritumomab tiuxetan and high-dose chemotherapy in patients with non-Hodgkin's lymphoma. *J Clin Oncol.* 2008;26(1):90-95.

[88] Gopal AK, Rajendran JG, Petersdorf SH, et al. High-dose chemo-radioimmunotherapy with autologous stem cell support for relapsed mantle cell lymphoma. *Blood.* 2002;99(9):3158-3162.

[89] Shanbhag S, Smith MR, Emmons RV. Tackling mantle cell lymphoma (MCL): Potential benefit of allogeneic stem cell transplantation. *Stem Cells Cloning.* 2010;3:93-102.

[90] Maris MB, Sandmaier BM, Storer BE, et al. Allogeneic hematopoietic cell transplantation after fludarabine and 2 Gy total body irradiation for relapsed and refractory mantle cell lymphoma. *Blood.* 2004;104 (12):3535-3542.

[91] Robinson SP, Sureda A, Canals C, Sr., et al. Identification of Prognostic Factors Predicting the Outcome of Reduced Intensity Allogeneic Stem Cell Transplantation in Mantle Cell Lymphoma. An Analysis from the Lymphoma Working Party of the EBMT. 2008.

[92] Dietrich S, Boumendil A, Finel H, et al. Outcome and prognostic factors in patients with mantle-cell lymphoma relapsing after autologous stem-cell transplantation: a retrospective study of the European Group for Blood and Marrow Transplantation (EBMT). *Ann Oncol.* 2014;25(5):1053-1058.

[93] Khan WN. Regulation of B lymphocyte development and activation by Bruton's tyrosine kinase. *Immunol Res.* 2001;23(2-3):147-156.

[94] Rinaldi A, Kwee I, Taborelli M, et al. Genomic and expression profiling identifies the B-cell associated tyrosine kinase Syk as a possible therapeutic target in mantle cell lymphoma. *Br J Haematol.* 2006;132(3):303-316.

[95] Friedberg JW, Sharman J, Sweetenham J, et al. Inhibition of Syk with fostamatinib disodium has significant clinical activity in non-Hodgkin lymphoma and chronic lymphocytic leukemia. *Blood.* 2010;115(13):2578-2585.

[96] Hoellenriegel J, Meadows SA, Sivina M, et al. The phosphoinositide 3'-kinase delta inhibitor, CAL-101, inhibits B-cell receptor signaling and chemokine networks in chronic lymphocytic leukemia. *Blood.* 2011;118(13):3603-3612.

[97] Lannutti BJ, Meadows SA, Herman SE, et al. CAL-101, a p110delta selective phosphatidylinositol-3-kinase inhibitor for the treatment of B-cell malignancies, inhibits PI3K signaling and cellular viability. *Blood.* 2011;117(2):591-594.

[98] Meadows SA, Vega F, Kashishian A, et al. PI3Kdelta inhibitor, GS-1101 (CAL-101), attenuates pathway signaling, induces apoptosis, and overcomes signals from the microenvironment in cellular models of Hodgkin lymphoma. *Blood.* 2012;119(8):1897-1900.

[99] Liu N, Rowley BR, Bull CO, et al. BAY 80-6946 is a highly selective intravenous PI3K inhibitor with potent p110alpha and p110delta activities in tumor cell lines and xenograft models. *Mol Cancer Ther.* 2013;12(11):2319-2330.

[100] Kahl BS, Spurgeon SE, Furman RR, et al. A phase 1 study of the PI3Kdelta inhibitor idelalisib in patients with relapsed/refractory mantle cell lymphoma (MCL). *Blood.* 2014;123(22):3398-3405.

[101] Preliminary results of a phase II study of single agent Bay 80-6946, a Novel PI3K inhibitor, in patients with relapsed/refractory, indolent or aggressive lymphoma. *Clin Adv Hematol Oncol.* 2014;12(2 Suppl 5):14-16.

[102] Temsirolimus: CCI 779, CCI-779, cell cycle inhibitor-779. *Drugs R D.* 2004;5(6):363-367.

[103] Witzig TE, Geyer SM, Ghobrial I, et al. Phase II trial of single-agent temsirolimus (CCI-779) for relapsed mantle cell lymphoma. *J Clin Oncol.* 2005;23(23):5347-5356.

[104] Ansell SM, Inwards DJ, Rowland KM, Jr., et al. Low-dose, single-agent temsirolimus for relapsed mantle cell lymphoma: a phase 2 trial in the North Central Cancer Treatment Group. *Cancer.* 2008;113(3):508-514.

[105] Hess G, Herbrecht R, Romaguera J, et al. Phase III study to evaluate temsirolimus compared with investigator's choice therapy for the treatment of relapsed or refractory mantle cell lymphoma. *J Clin Oncol.* 2009;27(23):3822-3829.

[106] Ansell SM, Tang H, Kurtin PJ, et al. Temsirolimus and rituximab in patients with relapsed or refractory mantle cell lymphoma: a phase 2 study. *Lancet Oncol.* 2011;12(4):361-368.

[107] Davids MS, Seymour JF, Gerecitano JF, et al. Updated results of a phase I first-in-human study of the BCL-2 inhibitor ABT-199 (GDC-0199) in patients with relapsed/refractory non-Hodgkin lymphoma (NHL). 2013.

[108] Alduaij W, Ivanov A, Honeychurch J, et al. Novel type II anti-CD20 monoclonal antibody (GA101) evokes homotypic adhesion and actin-

dependent, lysosome-mediated cell death in B-cell malignancies. *Blood.* 2011;117(17):4519-4529.

[109] Morschhauser FA, Cartron G, Thieblemont C, et al. Obinutuzumab (GA101) monotherapy in relapsed/refractory diffuse large b-cell lymphoma or mantle-cell lymphoma: results from the phase II GAUGUIN study. *J Clin Oncol.* 2013;31(23):2912-2919.

[110] Barth MJ, Pendurti G, Tsai P-C, et al. Ofatumumab (OFA) Is a Novel Anti-CD20 Monoclonal Antibody (mAb) with Improved Anti-Tumor Activity in Vitro and in Vivo in Mantle Cell Lymphoma (MCL) Pre-Clinical Models. 2012.

[111] Hunstig F, Hammersen J, Kunert C, et al. Complete remission after treatment with single-agent ofatumumab in a patient with high-risk leukemic mantle-cell lymphoma. *J Clin Oncol.* 2013;31(19):e312-315.

[112] Magni M, Di Nicola M, Carlo-Stella C, et al. Safety, Tolerability and Activity of Ofatumumab, Bendamustine and Dexamethasone Combination As First-Line Treatment of Mantle-Cell Lymphoma in the Elderly: A Multicenter Study. 2011.

[113] Leonard JP, LaCasce AS, Smith MR, et al. Selective CDK4/6 inhibition with tumor responses by PD0332991 in patients with mantle cell lymphoma. *Blood.* 2012;119(20):4597-4607.

[114] Ogura M, Ando K, Suzuki T, et al. A multicentre phase II study of vorinostat in patients with relapsed or refractory indolent B-cell non-Hodgkin lymphoma and mantle cell lymphoma. *Br J Haematol.* 2014;165(6):768-776.

[115] Evens AM, Vose JM, Harb W, et al. A Phase II Multicenter Study of the Histone Deacetylase Inhibitor (HDACi) Abexinostat (PCI-24781) in Relapsed/Refractory Follicular Lymphoma (FL) and Mantle Cell Lymphoma (MCL). 2012.

[116] Rolland D, Ribrag V, Haioun C, et al. Phase II trial and prediction of response of single agent tipifarnib in patients with relapsed/refractory mantle cell lymphoma: a Groupe d'Etude des Lymphomes de l'Adulte trial. *Cancer Chemother Pharmacol.* 2010;65(4):781-790.

[117] Palanca-Wessels MC, Flinn IW, Sehn LH, et al. A Phase I Study of the Anti-CD79b Antibody-Drug Conjugate (ADC) DCDS4501A Targeting CD79b in Relapsed or Refractory B-Cell Non-Hodgkin's Lymphoma (NHL). 2012.

In: Mantle Cell Lymphoma
Editor: Charles L. Schmidt

ISBN: 978-1-63482-363-0


*Chapter 3*

# Targeted Drugs in the Treatment of Mantle Cell Lymphoma

***Piotr Smolewski*[1], *Magdalena Witkowska*[1,2] *and Tadeusz Robak*[2,*]**
[1]Department of Experimental Hematology,
Medical University of Lodz, Poland
[2]Department of Hematology, Medical University of Lodz,
Copernicus Memorial Hospitall, Lodz, Poland

## Abstract

Mantle cell lymphoma (MCL) is a type of non-Hodgkin lymphoma characterized by an indolent histologic picture but an aggressive clinical course. The cytogenetic marker of MCL is chromosomal translocation t(11;14) (q13; q32), with expression of cyclin D1. As MCL remains incurable, modification of its treatment represents an important challenge. The introduction of rituximab, more intensive chemotherapy and the increasing use of autologous stem cell transplant (ASCT) in first remission has results in some improvement in the survival of MCL patients. Recently, several targeted agents have shown promising activity in MCL, of which lenalidomide, proteasome inhibitors or m-TOR

* Correspondence to: Prof. Tadeusz Robak, Department of Hematology, Medical University of Lodz, Copernicus Memorial Hospital, Ciolkowskiego 2, 93-510 Lodz, Poland.

inhibitor were found to be efficient in relapsed and refractory disease, even when used as a single agents. Moreover, B-cell receptor pathway inhibitors such as ibrutinib and idelalisib have also shown high activity, since abnormalities in this pathway are believed to be crucial in MCL pathogenesis. Similarly, histone deacetylase (HDAC) or cyclin-dependent kinase inhibitors have shown some promise in early phase trials. In this review we present the state of the art for emerging targeted therapies for MCL.

## Introduction

Mantle cell lymphoma (MCL) represents approximately 3-10% of non-Hodgkin lymphomas (NHL), and has increased in incidence over the past several decades [1, 2]. The clinical course is aggressive in most patients, although more indolent in others [3]. Most patients present advanced stage disease, with a trend towards extranodal, especially gastrointestinal, involvement. The majority of patients respond to initial therapy, but remission duration is typically short: ranging from 1.5 to 3 years [4, 5]. However, the prognosis in MCL is still poor due to aggressive clinical course, low sensitivity to standard chemotherapy, and high rates of relapse [6]. Median overall survival (OS) is 3 to 4 years. The clinical course is heterogeneous. Although some patients demonstrate a highly aggressive and rapid course, the disease has an indolent character in a small proportion of patients, who may survive more than 10 years, even without any treatment [6].

For several years, the CHOP (cyclophosphamide, doxorubicin, vincristine, prednisone) regimen was used as standard first line chemotherapy in MCL, although this was strengthened in the last decade by the addition of rituximab, a monoclonal anti-D20 antibody (R-CHOP regimen). Rituximab added to either chemotherapy or to preparative regimens prior to autologous stem cell transplantation (ASCT) has been shown to improve OS and progression free survival (PFS) in MCL patients [7-10].

The heterogenous course of the disease indicates the necessity for treatment individualization according to prognostic factors. The MCL prognostic index (MIPI) has already been developed based on data from clinical trials [11, 12]. Currently, first therapy for MCL is divided into modalities for younger patients, who may be eligible for ASCT, and older patients, who may be unfit for such an aggressive approach. In both types of upfront MCL therapy, two crucial agents are used, and one of them is rituximab.

# Upfront Treatment

## Aggressive Immunochemotherapy in Transplant-eligible MCL Patients

High-dose cytarabine was first exploited in this context as part of the dose-intense hyper-CVAD regimen (hyperfractionated cyclophosphamide, vincristine, doxorubicin, dexamethasone) with good results in single-arm, single-centre settings [12]. The addition of rituximab to this regimen gives extremely high CR rates of 87-92% [13, 14]. Another study found response rates to R-hyper CVAD/cytarabine and methotrexate to be high (72% complete remission, CR), however, 5-year failure-free survival responses of 46% and significant cytotoxicity were also noted [15].

The effective doses of high-dose cytarabine derived from these regimens were subsequently incorporated into other combination chemotherapies. The results of the Nordic MCL2 study [16] were far superior to the Nordic MCL1 trial, with the main differences between the two trials being the addition of rituximab and high-dose cytarabine in MCL2.

In the MCL Younger study, which evaluated alternating courses of R-CHOP and R-DHAP (rituximab, dexamethasone, cytarabine, cisplatin), followed by a high-dose cytarabine-containing conditioning regimen for ASCT, CR rates were significantly higher than those in observed in an arm with R-CHOP and conventional myeloablative conditioning [17]. This treatment was associated with long-term remission in several patients, especially in those with low and intermediate MIPI score [16]. Currently, as recommended by the European MCL Network, high dose cytarabine-containing induction and conditioning regimens such as R-CHOP alternating with R-DHAP, followed by ASCT consolidation should be considered for clinically fit patients with MCL younger than 60-65 years [17].

## Aggressive Therapy without Transplant Consolidation

An alternate regimen utilizing high-dose cytarabine and high-dose methotrexate in the absence of a transplant procedure has been investigated. In a single-center phase II study, 97 patients with MCL received R-hyper-CVAD alternating with R-MA (rituximab, high dose methotrexate, and cytarabine) [14, 19]. In a 10-year follow-up analysis, the initial CR rate was 87% and the median OS was not reached. Median time to treatment failure (TTF) was 4.6 years. Elevated beta-2 microglobulin and poor-risk IPI and MIPI were found to predict OS. Patients older than 65 years had significantly poorer OS and TTF, with worse hematological toxicity. A subsequent multicenter study of the same regimen prior to ASCT demonstrated worse toxicity than the single center study with lower response rates [20]. Other studies have also shown unacceptable degrees of myelosuppression and toxicity-related deaths when using modified R-hyper-CVAD in an elderly population [21]. This regimen can be considered in younger patients able to tolerate aggressive therapy but are otherwise unwilling or unable to undergo ASCT.

## Autologous Stem-cell Transplantation (ASCT)

In a randomized trial by Dreyling and et al. [22], patients who received ASCT in first remission demonstrated a better outcome than those receiving ASCT after relapse. In this study, previously untreated patients with advanced stage MCL were treated with CHOP-like induction chemotherapy. Patients with partial response (PR) or CR were then randomized to receive either myeloablative radio chemotherapy followed by ASCT vs. two more cycles of CHOP-like consolidation followed by interferon-alpha maintenance and ASCT at relapse. After a median follow-up of 25 months, patients who received ASCT in first remission had median PFS of 39 months, compared with 17 months for patients with IFN-α maintenance and ASCT at relapse. Although authors did not find significant differences in OS, ASCT in first remission may represent an optimal treatment for eligible patients after aggressive induction with rituximab and high-dose cytarabine-based regimens [23, 24].

Both the Nordic MCL2 trial mentioned above and the Groupe d'Etude des Lymphomes de l'Adulte (GELA) evaluated CHOP and high dose cytarabine regimens plus rituximab followed by ASCT [16, 25]. In the GELA trial, this therapy showed long-term efficacy with a median event free survival (EFS) of 83 months and a 5-year OS rate of 75% (median follow-up of 67 months).

Rituximab was also found to be effective in stem cell purging before ASCT after high-dose sequential chemotherapy, with long-term remissions noted at a 54-month follow-up examination. OS and EFS rates were also found to be 89% and 79%, respectively [26].

## Treatment of Unfit and Elderly MCL Patients

Although ASCT remains a treatment option both in first remission and at relapse, it is not curative in the majority of patients with MCL, and many are not ASCT candidates due to age and comorbidities. The disease presents most commonly in elderly patients not eligible for transplant. Thus, in this group or in younger patients with a poor performance status or comorbidities, treatment should be less aggressive.

The German Study Group of Indolent Lymphomas performed a randomized phase III clinical trial comparing the combination of R-bendamustine (BR) with R-CHOP [29]. BR was associated with significantly longer progression free survival (PFS), but with less toxicity.

Another study evaluated the response to BR vs R-CVP (rituximab, cyclophosphamide, vincristine, prednisone) or R-CHOP in 419 patients with untreated NHL. Although BR showed a higher CR rate among MCL patients (51% vs 24%), more side effects were also noted [28]. Despite this, BR is recommended as upfront therapy in elderly patients or for patients who may not eligible for more aggressive therapy.

## Rituximab Maintenance

Rituximab maintenance prolongs response duration after R in combination with chemotherapy, with no effect on OS [29, 30]. The MCL Elderly study by Dreyling et al., [31] which confirmed the value of adding rituximab to chemotherapy regimens, is currently examining whether maintenance rituximab will be of benefit. The available data from this study suggests that rituximab maintenance may increase overall response rates (ORR) and OS, particularly following R-CHOP, as compared with rituximab, fludarabine, cyclofosfamide, (R-FC) as initial therapy [32]. Elderly patients may also benefit from BR with maintenance rituximab following induction therapy. While standard chemoimmunotherapy provides high ORR, the responses are not durable. Despite improved PFS rates with BR therapy and prolonged remission durations reported with rituximab maintenance, no plateau is observed in PFS with any of the examined approaches [33].

Although standard immunochemotherapy provides high ORR, there is no proven curative treatment for MCL patients. According to recent investigations, MCL is highly sensitive to novel therapies that may in the near future become useful adjuncts to standard regimens.

# Targeted Treatment in Resistant/Relapsed MCL Patients

There are several mechanisms of cell cycle or cell survival impaired in MCL (Figure 1). Toward this end a number of biologically targeted strategies are under investigations.

**Table 1. Novel agents in mantle cell lymphoma**

| Agent | Drug class | n | Disease Status | med. age (years) | OS | ORR (%) | PFS (months) | Lead Author |
|---|---|---|---|---|---|---|---|---|
| Ibrutinib | Btk inhibitor | 111 | R/R | 68 | NR | 68 | 13.9 | Wang et al. [101] |
| Idelalisib | PI3K inhibitor | 40 | R/R | 69 | 22% 1 year | 40 | 3.7 | Kahl et al. [104] |
| Fostamatinib | Syk inhibitor | 9 | R/R | - | NR | 11 | 3.8 | Friedberg et al. [109] |
| Alvocidib | CDK inhibitor | 17 | R/R | 66 | - | 18 | > 1 year | Leonard et al. [93] |
| Everolimus | mTOR inhibitor | 35 | R/R | 70 | 12 months | 38 | 6.5 | Witzig et al. [113] |
| Bortezomib | proteasome inhibitor | 11 | R/R | 65 | 23.5 months | 69 | 6.7 | Goy et al. [115] |
| Lenalidomide | proteasome inhibitor | 57 | R/R | 68 | NR | 35 | 8.8 | Zinzani et al. [120] |
| Avastin + R-CHOP | anti-VEGF mAb | 11 | untreated | 60 | 82% 3 years | 82 | 18 | Certo et al. [128] |

n= number of patients, OS = overall survival, ORR = objective response rate, - = not evaluated, NR = not reached, R/ = relapsed or refractory, PFS = progression free survival, PI3K = phosphoinositol-3 kinase, Btk = Bruton's tyrosine kinase, Syk = spleen tyrosine kinase, CDK = Cyclin Dependent Kinase, mTOR = mammalian target of rapamycin, VEGF = vascular endothelial growth factor, mAb= monoclonal antibody

## Monoclonal Antibodies

Following the success of rituximab, various anti-CD20 monoclonal antibodies (mAbs) have been studied in B cell lymphoma including MCL. Attempts have been made to engineer novel regimens to enhance either antibody-dependent cell-mediated cytotoxicity (ADCC) or complement activation to strengthen their cytotoxic activity [34, 35]. Although little data specific for MCL exists, antibody-drug conjugates are still an active area of investigation.

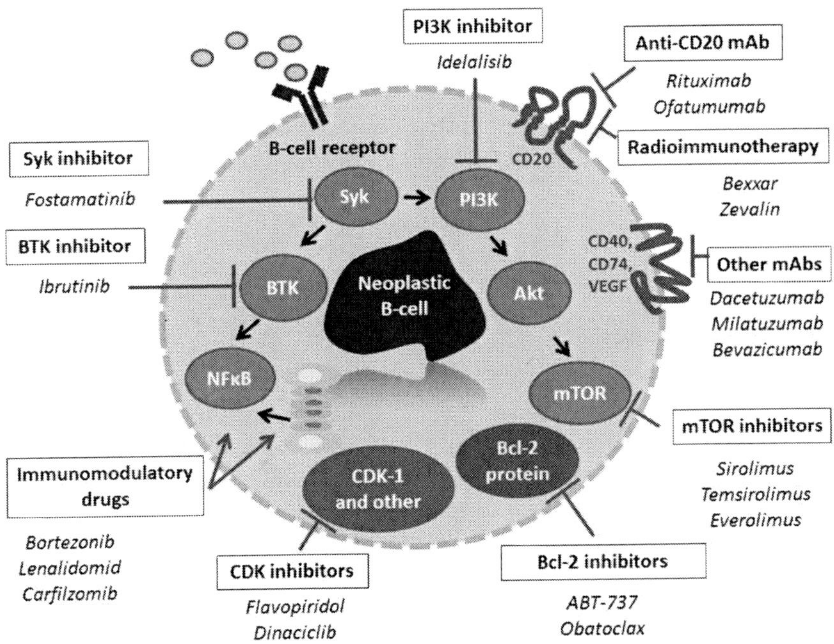


Abbreviations: PI3K - phosphoinositol-3 kinase; mAb – monoclonal antibody; mTOR – mammalian target of rapamycin; CDK - cyclin dependent kinase; BTK - Bruton's tyrosine kinase; Syk - spleen tyrosine kinase; BCR – B-cell receptor.

Figure 1. The targets for biological treatment in mantle cell lymphoma.

CD40 is a type-1 transmembrane protein of the tumor necrosis factor (TNF) receptor superfamily, expressed on B cells and the majority of B-cell malignancies including NHL, MM, and chronic lymphocytic leukemia [36]. Dacetuzumab, a humanized monoclonal mAb against CD40, has been investigated in a phase I clinical trial for patients with relapsed and refractory B-cell lymphomas including MCL [37]. In the evaluated group, six patients (12%) demonstrated objective responses to the studied drug and 13 additional patients (26%) had stable disease (SD). A PR was observed in 1 out of 10 patients with the MCL subtype enrolled in this study. Most side effects were grade 1 or 2, with a safe toxicity profile.

Another mAb which has been investigated in MCL is milatuzumab, a humanized anti-CD74 mAb. CD74 expression is rather limited in normal cells, but it was found to be overexpressed in more than 85% of NHL [39]. CD74 activation is believed to mediate proliferative and prosurvival signaling and can activate the PI3K/m TOR/Akt pathway, leading to increased malignant B-cell survival. In an *in vitro* study, Alinari et al. report enhanced cell death in MCL cell lines by a combination of rituximab and milatuzumab, two mAbs which are known to target distinct antigens and potentially signal through different pathways [40]. Hence, further clinical evaluations of the use of this milatuzumab and rituximab combination in treatment of MCL are required.

## Radio Immunotherapy

Radio immunotherapy (RIT) links a mAb with a radioactive agent in order to deliver radiation directly to the neoplastic B-cell and immediate surroundings, while minimizing systemic radiation exposure. Currently, there are two approved RIT agents for use in B-cell lymphoma: $^{131}$I-tositumomab (Bexxar) and $^{90}$Y-ibritumomab tiuxetan (Zevalin), both target CD20. Unfortunately the data regarding the efficacy of RIT treatment in MCL is limited.

In a phase II trial of RIT with Zevalin in relapsed and refractory MCL, the median ORR was found to be 31% with a median follow-up of 22 months, median OS was 21 months and EFS was 6 months [40]. Importantly, patients were heavily pretreated with a median of three prior chemotherapy lines, including 22 who had previously received HyperCVAD. The majority of toxicities observed in this study was primarily haematological, transient, and reversible. In a trial by Zelenetz et al. [41], sequential therapy of RIT with Bexxar followed by CHOP chemotherapy for patients with newly diagnosed advanced stage MCL was investigated. While the median ORR in the RIT group was 83% (CR/CRu 46%; PR 38%) among the twenty-four patients treated in the trial, the ORR rose to 86% for the twenty-one patients who continued to consolidation with CHOP. It can be seen that a much higher response rate can be observed when RIT is used as initial therapy and when a heavily pretreated group of relapsed and refractory patients is examined. MCL is a fairly radiosensitive lymphoma type and RIT can be an integrated part of future treatment in combination with other novel agents.

## Cyclin Dependent Kinase Inhibition

Considering the crucial role of cyclin D1 in the pathogenesis of MCL, inhibition of this pathway should be a logical strategy for target specific treatment. However, no specific inhibitor of cyclin D1 is currently available for patients with an MCL diagnosis. Cyclin Dependent Kinase (CDK) is an enzyme that complexes with cyclin D1, ultimately promoting proliferation of normal and neoplastic cells. Inhibition of this kinase can be accomplished by inhibition of its catalytic partners, CDK4 and CDK6: isoforms that led to retinoblastoma protein phosphorylation blockage, resulting in cell cycle arrest. Alvocidib (flavopiridol) was found to be a potential CDK9 inhibitor, recently widely investigated in clinical trials [42-44]. A phase Ib study of flavopirydol in 17 relapsed and refractory MCL patients found the median PFS over 1 year to be 29.4% (5 of the 17 patients) and the median ORR 18% [45]. Grade III and IV adverse events (AEs), including neutropenia and thrombocytopenia, were common, but easily controlled. Unfortunately, clinical trials found the anticancer activity of flavopiridol in monotherapy to be marginal. Some ongoing clinical studies exploring flavopiridol in combination with histone deacetylase inhibitors, proteasome inhibitors, and other conventionally used cytotoxic agents are ongoing [46-47]. Nowadays, more specific or potent CDK inhibitors are also under investigation. PD0332991 is a specific, well-tolerated inhibitor of CDK4 and CDK6, with strong anticancer activity [48]. Another novel inhibitor of CDK1, -2, -5, and -9 is SCH727965 (dinaciclib). It has already revealed stronger anticancer activity and an improved therapeutic index than flavopiridol in laboratory models based on both hematologic malignancies and solid tumors [49].

However, as no preliminary data has shown any dramatic response of MCL to these CDK inhibitors, there must be other deregulated pathway that is responsible for the growth and survival of MCL cells.

## Inhibitors of B-Cell Receptor Signaling

In addition to pathognomonic t (11;14) resulting in aberrant expression of cyclin D1, hyperactivity of the B-cell receptor (BCR) signaling pathway was also discovered to contribute to the pathogenesis of MCL [50]. This pathway and its associated protein-tyrosine kinases play a critical role in the development, proliferation, and survival of both normal and neoplastic B-cells [51]. Novel agents that inhibit various components of the BCR pathway are currently under investigation in clinical trials, including inhibitors of phosphoinositol-3 kinase (PI3K), Bruton's tyrosine kinase (Btk) and spleen tyrosine kinase (Syk) [52].

Ibrutinib, an irreversible and selective Btk inhibitor formerly called PCI-32765, has already demonstrated significant therapeutic potential in various types of B-cell malignancies, including MCL. In a multicenter, phase II trial by Wang et al., 111 patients with relapsed or refractory MCL were treated with oral ibrutinib at a daily dose of 560 mg [53]. The median age was 68 years, 86% was intermediate or high risk according to MIPI score, with the median of 3 prior lines of treatment. Ibrutinib demonstrated significant efficacy, with an ORR of 68% (CR- 21%), the estimated median PFS was 13.9 months, and the median OS was not reached. In another recent study evaluating the activity of ibrutinib in patients with relapsed or refractory B-cell malignancies, 9 patients with MCL were included [54]. The median ORR was 78% in MCL patients with a median PFS of 13.5 months in all subtypes of lymphoma. The most common side effects were grade I and II including fatigue, diarrhea, dizziness and peripheral edema. Grade III and IV AEs occurred rarely, with the most common diarrhea, rash, neutropenic fever, and abdominal pain.

The first-in-class agent that could selectively inhibit the delta isoform of PI3K was idelalisib (CAL-101). It was discovered that the PI3K pathway is constitutively activated in the majority of B-cell malignant diseases, including MCL. This pathway is responsible for the growth, promotion and prolongation of cancer cell survival [55]. A phase I study was performed with 40 patients with relapsed or refractory MCL, the median age being 69 years, with a median of 4 prior therapies received [56]. The median ORR was 40%, with CR achieved in 2 of 40 patients (5%). The median PFS was 3.7 months and 1-year OS was 22%. The most common grade $\geq 3$ side effects were diarrhea, nausea, rash, decreased appetite and alanine transaminase or aspartate transaminase elevations.

Syk represents another therapeutic target for MCL due to a crucial role in the BCR signaling pathway. Fostamatinib disodium, a novel Syk inhibitor is one of the first compounds designed and developed to inhibit the BCR pathway. Syk plays a key role in BCR-dependent B-cell activation and immunoglobulin secretion. It has already demonstrated a good response in patients with relapsed B-cell malignancies in recent clinical trials [57]. Fostamatinib was the first clinically investigated oral Syk inhibitor in patients with relapsed or refractory B-cell lymphoma as well as different solid tumors [58-60]. In a phase I/II clinical trial investigating patients with relapsed or refractory B-cell lymphomas, 9 patients with MCL were evaluated [61]. The median ORR for MCL patients was 11% (1/9 patients) with median PFS 3.8 months. Therapy was generally well tolerated, with side effects including diarrhea, cytopenias, easy fatigue, hypertension and nausea.

Further studies are needed to establish inhibition of BCR signaling pathway as a clinically important therapeutic target in patients with MCL diagnosis.

## Mammalian Target of Rapamycin Inhibitors

Recently, inhibitors of the mammalian target of rapamycin (mTOR) are promising agents that may be successfully used for lymphoma treatment. Elevated mTOR activity is observed in the great majority of neoplastic cells, including hematological malignancies [62]. Targeting mTOR with specific mTOR inhibitors is a novel anticancer approach that may affect the survival of relapsed and refractory lymphoma patients [63]. The first drug investigated in clinical studies was macrolide antibiotic rapamycin (sirolimus). Its main mechanisms of action comprise cell arrest in the $G_1$ phase of the cell cycle and apoptosis [64]. Moreover, it has antiproliferative and antiangiogenic effects. Recently, two newer rapamycin analogs, everolimus and temsirolimus, have been extensively evaluated in clinical trials. Everolimus, an oral mTOR inhibitor, was widely evaluated by in relapsed and refractory MCL both in phase II and phase III clinical trials. A phase II clinical trial by Witzig et al. [65] included thirty-five MCL patients with a median age of 70 years, who had received a median of three prior therapies, 91% of whom were stage 4. The ORR was found to be 38% (with 3% CR, 35% PR), the median PFS was 6.5 months and the duration of response for the 13 responders was 6.9 months. The most frequent hematologic toxicity was thrombocytopenia (71% grade 3, 11% grade 4).

In the phase III multicenter, open-label study, 162 patients with relapsed or refractory MCL received one of two temsirolimus doses (higher-175/75-mg and lower- 175/25-mg) or the best investigator's choice (for e.g., gemcitabine, fludarabine, chlorambucil, or cladribine) [66]. In this trial, the median PFS was 4.8, 3.4, and 1.9 months for the temsirolimus higher dose, temsirolimus lower dose and the investigator's choice group, respectively. It was observed that patients treated with temsirolimus 175/75-mg had significantly longer PFS than those treated with investigator's choice therapy (P = 0.0009) and those treated with lower dose of temsirolimus (P = 0.0618). The median ORR was

22% for the higher temsirolimus dose compared with 2% in the investigator's choice group. The median OS for the higher temsirolimus dose was 12.8 months and 9.7 months for the investigator's choice group. The most frequently occurring grade 3 or 4 side-effects in the temsirolimus groups were thrombocytopenia, anemia, neutropenia and asthenia.

These results led to the approval of temsirolimus in Europe. mTOR inhibitors are not only highly active regiments in relapsed and refractory MCL but are also well tolerated.

## Immunomodulatory Drugs

Bortezomib, a specific proteasome inhibitor, was originally developed for the treatment of relapsed and refractory multiple myeloma (MM), and still is one of the most effective therapies available for those patients. Although it is another novel regimen recently approved by the FDA for the treatment of relapsed and refractory MCL, its exact mechanism is not fully understood. In the PINNACLE multicenter, phase II clinical trial, bortezomib activity was evaluated as a single agent in patients with relapsed or refractory MCL [67]. Bortezomib was administered subcutaneously at 1.3 mg/m$^2$ on days 1, 4, 8, 11 in a 21-day cycle. The median OS was 23.5 months, and 35.4 months in the responding group of patients, with a manageable toxicity profile. Median time to progression (TTP) was 6.7 months and median time to next therapy (TTNT) was 7.4 months. Another an international phase I/II study, a clinical trial investigated the addition of botrezomib to standard R-CHOP therapy [68]. In this study, 36 previously untreated MCL patients with generally unfavorable MIPI scores, 28% intermediate-risk and 39% high-risk, with an average age of 66 years were evaluated. The evaluable ORR was 81%, with a 2 year PFS of 44 %, and 2 year OS of 86%. The results of randomized studies indicate that bortezomib is a safe and highly-effective regimen in patients with relapsed and refractory MCL.

Another second generation immunomodulatory drug recently investigated in patients with MCL is lenalidomide: a synthetic derivative of thalidomide with a different cytotoxic effect. It is already approved in MM [69] and myelodysplastic syndrome [70]. The anticancer mechanism is complex and is composed of direct cell cycle-arresting effects which exert a proapoptotic influence on cancer cells. Moreover, it influences the physical and functional interaction with the tumor microenvironment and exerts a pleiotropic immunostimulatory effect [71]. Recently, the potential for lenalidomide to be used as a single agent in relapsed and refractory MCL patients was evaluated in two multicenter phase II clinical trials [72, 73]. The phase II NHL-003 trial investigated 57 advanced-stage MCL patients with a median of three prior treatment lines [72]. The observed ORR was 35%, the median PFS was 8.8 months and the median duration of response (DOR) was 16.3 months. The OS has not yet been reached. The most common side-effects, including neutropenia (46%), thrombocytopenia (30%), and anemia (13%) were manageable in the majority of patients. Another multicenter phase II study EMERGE examined the safety and efficacy of lenalidomide in patients who had relapsed or were refractory to bortezomib [73]. A total of 134 patients were enrolled to this study with a median age of 67 years and a median four prior treatment lines. The ORR was 28% with a median PFS of 4.0 months and median OS of 19.0 months. The observed side effects were similar to those seen in a previous study with a safe profile.

Data from phase I/II clinical studies demonstrates that rituximab and lenalidomide exert strongly synergic activity when used in combination in relapsed and refractory MCL patients [74]. Fifty-two patients (14 in phase I and 44 in phase II) were enrolled in this single-arm, open-label trial. Among the 44 patients incorporated in the phase II study, the ORR was 57% (CR-36%, PR 20%) with a median OS of 24.3 months and median PFS of 11.1 months. The majority of patients reported prior exposure to rituximab. According to this study, oral lenalidomide was found to be both well tolerated and effective for the heavily pretreated group of MCL patients.

Another newer generation proteasome inhibitor, carfilzomib, is currently under investigation in clinical trials. Carfilzomib is a second-generation proteasome inhibitor that irreversibly and preferentially targets the chymotrypsin-like activity of the 20S core proteasome and immunoproteasome [75]. It was recently discovered that the ORR of carfilzomib, when used as a single agent in patients with relapsed MM, ranges from 50% to 60% with minimal neuropathy [76, 77]. However, data on the clinical activity of carfilzomib in MCL is currently extremely limited. Nevertheless, in future we anticipate further preclinical studies investigating the use of carfilzomib in combination with the histone deacetylase inhibitor vorinostat in B-cell and T-cell lymphomas based on the strong synergy of these drugs observed in MCL [78].

## Anti-VEGF Monoclonal Antibody

The tumour microenvironment and the presence of tumor-associated angiogenesis is very important in oncogenesis. It has already been observed that a high pretreatment serum vascular endothelial growth factor (VEGF) concentration is associated with poor outcome in B-cell lymphoma [79]. The novel agent bevacizumab (Avastin, Genentech) is a recombinant, humanized mAb directed against all isoforms of VEGF. Although bevacizumab is not active as a single agent, it has been found to enhance the efficacy of standard chemotherapy in lymphoma patients with high expression of VEGF [79]. Recently, a phase II trial data evaluating the addition of bevacizumab to the standard R-CHOP regimen in 11 previously untreated MCL patients were published [80]. The median ORR was 82% with a 36% CR, the median PFS was 18 months and 3-year OS rate was 82%. Beyond the standard side effects connected with R-CHOP treatment, only left ventricular dysfunction was observed as grade 3 AE. To conclude, the addition of bevacizumab to the standard R-CHOP regimen unfortunately does not appear to significantly improve efficacy compared to R-CHOP used alone.

## BCL-2 Inhibitors

Overexpression of the prosurvival Bcl-2 family members (Bcl-2, Bcl-xL, and Mcl-1) is known to be commonly associated with cancer development, progression, and chemoresistance [81]. Consequently, Bcl-2 and its prosurvival homologues are attractive targets for therapeutic intervention. One new therapeutic approach is to induce apoptosis via the intrinsic pathway by antagonizing the antiapoptotic Bcl-2 family proteins. This approach is prompted by numerous studies showing that the antiapoptotic protein Bcl-2 is constitutively overexpressed in MCL and plays a major role in drug resistance [82, 83]. These findings highlight the potential role of Bcl-2–targeted therapy in MCL patients. ABT-737 is a new compound that selectively binds with high affinity to Bcl-2 and Bcl-xL, displaces proapoptotic BH3-only from Bcl-2 or Bcl-xL, and leads to activation of Bax and Bak and downstream caspases [84]. Recent studies have shown that ABT-737 is effective as a single agent against both leukemia and lymphoma cell lines, including MCL cell lines, both *in vitro* and *in vivo* [85, 86]. Clinical studies involving Bcl2-inhibitors such as ABT-737 are still ongoing, as well as others including obatoclax and AT-10.

# References

[1] Zhou Y., Wang H., Fang W., Romaguer J. E., Zhang Y. et al., Incidence trends of mantle *Cancer*. 2008; 113:791-8.

[2] Chandran R., Gardiner S. K., Simon M., Spurgeon S. E. Survival trends in mantle cell lymphoma in the United States over sixteen years 1992-2007. *Leuk Lymphoma* 2012; 53:1488-1493.

[3] Martin P., Chadburn A., Christos P., Weil K., Furman R. R. et al., Outcome of deferred initial therapy *J Clin Oncol*. 2009; 27:1209-13.

[4] Vose J. M. Mantle cell lymphoma: 2012 update on diagnosis, risk-stratification, and clinical management. *Am J Hematol* 2012; 87:605-609.

[5] Ruan J., Coleman M., Leonard J. P. Management of relapsed mantle cell lymphoma: still a treatment challenge. *Oncology* 2009; 23:683-690.

[6] Cortelazzo S., Ponzoni M., Ferreri A. J., Dreyling M. Mantle cell lymphoma. *Crit Rev Oncol Hematol*. 2012; 82:78-101.

[7] Thieblemont C., Antal D., Lacotte-Thierry L., Delwail V., Espinouse D., et al., Chemotherapy with rituximab *Cancer*. 200; 104:1434-41.

[8] Herold M. et al., Bendamustine, vincristine and prednisone (BOP) vs cyclophosphamide, vincristine and prednisone (COP) in advanced indolent non-Hodgkin's lymphoma and mantle cell lymphoma; results of a randomized phase III trial (OSHO# 19). *Cancer Res Clin Oncol*. 2006; 132:105-12.

[9] Lenz G., Dreyling M., Hoster E., Wörmann B., Dührsen U. et al., Immunochemotherapy with rituximab and cyclophosphamide, doxorubicin, vincristine, and prednisone significantly improves response and time to treatment failure, but not long-term outcome in patients with previously untreated mantle cell lymphoma: results of a prospective randomized trial of the German Low Grade Lymphoma Study Group (GLSG). *J Clin Oncol*. 2005; 23:1984-92.

[10] Forstpointner R., Unterhalt M., Dreyling M., Böck H. P., Repp R., German Low Grade Lymphoma Study Group (GLSG). Maintenance therapy with rituximab leads to a significant prolongation of response duration after salvage therapy with a combination of rituximab, fludarabine, cyclophosphamide, and mitoxantrone (R-FCM) in patients with recurring and refractory follicular and mantle cell lymphomas: results of a prospective randomized study of the German Low Grade Lymphoma Study Group (GLSG). *Blood*. 2006; 108: 4003-8.

[11] Hoster E., Dreyling M., Klapper W., Gisselbrecht C., van Hoof A. et al., German Low Grade Lymphoma Study Group (GLSG); European Mantle Cell Lymphoma Network. A new prognostic index (MIPI) for patients with advanced-stage mantle *Blood.* 2008; 111:558-65.

[12] Van de Schans S. A., Janssen-Heijnen M. L., Nijziel M. R., Steyerberg E. W., van Spronsen D. J. Validation, revision and extension of the Mantle Cell Lymphoma International Prognostic Index in a population-based setting. *Haematologica.* 2010; 95:1503-1509.

[13] Khouri I. F., Romaguera J., Kantarjian H., Palmer J. L., Pugh W. C. et al., Hyper-CVAD and high-dose methotrexate/cytarabine followed by stem-cell transplantation: an active regimen for aggressive mantle-cell lymphoma. *J Clin Oncol.* 1998; 16:3803-9.

[14] Ritchie D. S., Seymour J. F., Grigg A. P., Roberts A. W., Hoyt R. et al., The hyper-CVAD-rituximab chemotherapy programme followed by high-dose busulfan, melphalan and autologous stem cell transplantation produces excellent event-free survival in patients with previously untreated mantle cell lymphoma. *Ann Hematol.* 2007; 86:101-5.

[15] Romaguera J. E., Fayad L., Rodriguez M. A., Broglio K. R., Hagemeister F. B. et al., High rate of durable remissions after treatment of newly diagnosed aggressive mantle-cell lymphoma with rituximab plus hyper-CVAD alternating with rituximab plus high-dose methotrexate and cytarabine. *J Clin Oncol.* 2005; 23:7013-23.

[16] Merli F., Luminari S., Ilariucci F., Petrini M., Visco C. et al., Rituximab plus HyperCVAD alternating with high dose cytarabine and methotrexate for the initial treatment of patients with mantle cell lymphoma, a multicentre trial from Gruppo Italiano Studio Linfomi. *Br J Haematol.* 2012; 156:346-53.

[17] Geisler C. H., Kolstad A., Laurell A., Andersen N. S., Pedersen L. B. et al., Nordic Lymphoma Group. Long-term progression-free survival of mantle cell lymphoma after intensive front-line immunochemotherapy with *in vivo*-purged stem cell rescue: a nonrandomized phase 2 multicenter study by the Nordic Lymphoma Group. *Blood.* 2008; 112:2687-93.

[18] Hermine, O., Hoster, E., Walewski, J., Ribrag, V., Brousse, N. et al., Alternating courses of 3x CHOP and 3x DHAP plus rituximab followed by a high dose ARA-C containing myeloablative regimen and autologous stem cell transplantation (ASCT) Is superior to 6 courses CHOP plus rituximab followed by myeloablative radio chemotherapy and ASCT in mantle cell lymphoma: results of the MCL younger trial of

the European Mantle Cell Lymphoma network (MCL net). *Blood* (ASH Annual Meeting Abstracts), 2010; 116: 110.

[19] Geisler C. H., Kolstad A., Laurell A., Jerkeman M., Räty R. et al., Nordic Lymphoma Group. Nordic MCL2 trial *Br J Haematol.* 2012; 158:355-62.

[20] Romaguera J. E., Fayad L. E., Feng L., Hartig K., Weaver P. et al., Ten-year follow-up after intense chemoimmunotherapy with Rituximab-HyperCVAD alternating with Rituximab-high dose methotrexate/ cytarabine (R-MA) and without stem cell transplantation in patients with untreated aggressive mantle cell lymphoma. *Br J Haematol.* 2010; 150:200-8.

[21] Merli F., Luminari S., Ilariucci F., Petrini M., Visco C. et al., Rituximab plus HyperCVAD alternating with high dose cytarabine and methotrexate for the initial treatment of patients with mantle cell lymphoma, a multicentre trial from Gruppo Italiano Studio Linfomi. *Br J Haematol.* 2012; 156:346-53.

[22] Epner E. M. et al., A multi-center trial of hyperCVAD + rituxan in patients with newly diagnosed mantle cell lymphoma Presented at the American Society of Hematology annual meeting, Atlanta, GA, December 7-11, 2007. Abstract 387.

[23] Dreyling M., Lenz G., Hoster E., Van Hoof A., Gisselbrecht C. et al., Early consolidation by myeloablative radio chemotherapy followed by autologous stem cell transplantation in first remission significantly prolongs progression-free survival in mantle-cell lymphoma: results of a prospective randomized trial of the European MCL Network. *Blood* 2005; 105: 2677-84.

[24] Khouri I. F., Saliba R. M., Okoroji G. J., Acholonu S. A., Champlin R. E. Longterm follow-up of autologous stem cell transplantation in patients with diffuse mantle cell lymphoma in first disease remission: the prognostic value of beta2-microglobulin and the tumor score. *Cancer* 2003; 98:2630-5.

[25] Damon L. E., Johnson J. L., Niedzwiecki D., Cheson B. D., Hurd D. D. et al., Immunochemotherapy and autologous stem-cell transplantation for untreated patients with mantle-cell lymphoma: CALGB 59909. *J Clin Oncol* 2009; 27:6101-8.

[26] Delarue R., Haioun C., Ribrag V., Brice P., Delmer A. et al., Groupe d'Etude des Lymphomes de l'Adulte (GELA). CHOP and DHAP plus rituximab *Blood.* 2013; 121:48-53.

[27] Gianni A. M., Magni M., Martelli M., Di Nicola M., Carlo-Stella C. et al., Long-term remission *Blood.* 2003; 102:749-755.

[28] Kluin-Nelemans H. C., Hoster E., Hermine O., Walewski J., Trneny M. et al., Treatment of older patients with mantle *N Engl J Med.* 2012; 367:520-31.

[29] Flinn I. W., van der Jagt R., Kahl B. S., Wood P., Hawkins T. E. et al., Randomized trial *Blood* 2014; 123:2944-52.

[30] Forstpointner R., Unterhalt M., Dreyling M., Böck H. P., Repp R. et al., German Low Grade Lymphoma Study Group (GLSG). Maintenance therapy with rituximab leads to a significant prolongation of response duration after salvage therapy with a combination of rituximab, fludarabine, cyclophosphamide, and mitoxantrone (R-FCM) in patients with recurring and refractory follicular and mantle cell lymphomas: Results of a prospective randomized study of the German Low Grade Lymphoma Study Group (GLSG). *Blood.* 2006; 108:4003-8.

[31] Kahl B. S., Longo W. L., Eickhoff J. C., Zehnder J., Jones C., Blank J. et al., Wisconsin. Maintenance rituximab following induction chemoimmunotherapy may prolong progression-free survival in mantle cell lymphoma: a pilot study from the Wisconsin Oncology Network. *Ann Oncol.* 2006; 17: 1418-23.

[32] Dreyling M., Hoster E., Bea S., Hartmann E., Horn H. et al., European MCL Network. Update on the molecular pathogenesis and clinical treatment of Mantle Cell Lymphoma (MCL): minutes of the 9th European MCL Network conference. *Leuk* Lymphoma. 2010; 51:1612-22.

[33] Kluin-Nelemans, J. C, Hoster, E, Walewski, J, Stilgenbauer, S, Geisler, C. H, et al., R-CHOP versus R-FC followed by maintenance with rituximab versus interferon alfa: outcome of the first randomized trial for elderly patients with mantle cell lymphoma. *Blood (ASH Annual Meeting Abstracts),* 2011; 118, 439.

[34] Rummel M. J., Niederle N., Maschmeyer G., Banat G. A., von Grünhagen U. et al., Bendamustine plus rituximab versus CHOP plus rituximab as fi rst-line treatment for patients with indolent and mantle-cell lymphomas: an open label, multicentre, randomised, phase 3 non-inferiority trial. *Lancet* 2013; 38:1203-1210.

[35] Hagenbeek A., Gadeberg O., Johnson P., Pedersen L. M., Walewski J. et al., First clinical use of ofatumumab, a novel fully human anti-CD20 monoclonal antibody in relapsed or refractory follicular lymphoma: results of a phase 1/2 trial. *Blood* 2008; 111:5486-5495.

[36] Gruss H. J., Herrmann F., Gattei V. et al., CD40/CD40 ligand interactions in normal, reactive and malignant lympho-hematopoietic tissues. *Leuk Lymphoma* 1997:24:393-422.

[37] Advani R., Forero-Torres A., Furman R. R., Rosenblatt J. D., Younes A., Ren H., Harrop K., Whiting N., Drachman J. G. Phase I study of the humanized anti-CD40 monoclonal antibody dacetuzumab in refractory or recurrent non-Hodgkin's lymphoma. *J Clin Oncol* 2009; 27:4371-4377.

[38] Becker-Herman S., Arie G., Medvedovsky H., Kerem A., Shachar I. CD74 is a member of the regulated intramembrane proteolysis-processed protein family. *Mol Biol Cell.* 2005; 16:5061-9.

[39] Alinari L., Yu B., Christian B. A., Yan F., Shin J. et al., Combination anti-CD74 (milatuzumab) and anti-CD20 (rituximab) monoclonal antibody therapy has *in vitro* and *in vivo* activity in mantle cell lymphoma. *Blood* 117:4530-4541, 2011.

[40] Wang M., Oki Y. et al., Phase II study of yttrium-90-ibritumomab tiuxetan in patients with relapsed or refractory mantle cell lymphoma. *J Clin Oncol.* 2009; 27:5213-8.

[41] Zelenetz A. D. et al., Sequential radio immunotherapy with tositumomab/Iodine $I^{131}$ tositumomab followed by CHOP for mantle cell lymphoma demonstrates RIT can induce molecular remissions. *J Clin Oncol.* 2006; 24(18S):7560.

[42] Carlson B. A., Dubay M. M., Sausville E. A., Brizuela L., Worland P. J. Flavopiridol induces G1 arrest with inhibition of cyclin-dependent kinase (CDK) 2 and CDK4 in human breast carcinoma cells. *Cancer Res* 1996; 5 6:2973-8.

[43] Kaur G., Stetler-Stevenson M., Sebers S., Worland P., Sedlacek H., Myers C. et al., Growth inhibition with reversible cell cycle arrest of carcinoma cells by flavone L86-8275. *J Natl Cancer Inst* 1992; 84: 1736-40.

[44] Jayaraman A., Jamil K. Drug targets for cell cycle dysregulators in leukemogenesis: in silico docking studies. *PLoS* One. 2014; 9:e86310.

[45] Leonard J. P., La Casce A. S., Smith M. R., Noy A., Chirieac L. R. et al., Selective CDK4/6 inhibition with tumor responses by PD0332991 in patients with mantle cell lymphoma. *Blood.* 2012; 119:4597-607.

[46] Mason C. E., Di Liberto M., Huang X., Chiron D., Bretz J. et al., Mutation burden in CDKN2C, CDK1 and E2F2 is associated with differential response to targeting CDK4/CDK6 in combination with bortezomib in mantle cell lymphoma. *Blood* 2011; 118: 3738.

[47] Niesvizky R., Costa L. J., Haideri N. A., Hess G., Singhal S. et al., Preliminary results of a phase 2 study of PD 0332991 in combination with bortezomib and dexamethasone in patients with relapsed and refractory multiple myeloma. *Blood* 2011; 118:2940.

[48] Leonard J. P., La Casce A., Smith M. R., Noy A., Yap J. T. et al., Cdk4/6 inhibitor PD 0332991 demonstrates cell cycle inhibition via FLT-PET imaging and tissue analysis in patients with recurrent mantle cell lymphoma. *Blood* 2008; 112:264.

[49] Parry D., Guzi T., Shanahan F., Davis N., Prabhavalkar D. et al. Dinaciclib (SCH 727965), a novel and potent cyclin-dependent kinase inhibitor. *Mol Cancer Ther* 2010; 9:2344-53.

[50] Lenz G., Staudt L. M. Aggressive lymphomas. *N. Engl. J. Med.* 2010; 362: 1417-1429.

[51] Jares P., Colomer D., Campo E. Molecular pathogenesis of mantle cell lymphoma. *J Clin Invest* 2012; 122:3416-3423.

[52] Talar B., Czyż M. Rola szlaków sygnałowych TGF-β w nowotworach. *Postepy Hig Med Dosw* 2013; 67; 1008-1017.

[53] Wang M., Rule S. A., Martin P., Goy A., Auer R. et al., Targeting BTK with Ibrutinib in Relapsed or Refractory Mantle-Cell Lymphoma. *N Engl J Med* 2013; 369:507-516.

[54] Advani R. H., Buggy J. J., Sharman J. P., Smith S. M., Boyd T. et al., Bruton Tyrosine Kinase inhibitor ibrutinib (PCI-32765) has significant activity in patients with relapsed/refractory B-cell malignancies. *J Clin Oncol.* 2013; 31:88-94.

[55] Lo Piccolo J., Blumenthal G. M., Bernstein W. B., Dennis P. A. Targeting the PI3K/Akt/mTOR pathway: effective combinations and clinical considerations. *Drug Resist.* 2008; 11:32-50.

[56] Kahl B. S., Spurgeon S. E., Furman R. R., Flinn I. W., Coutre S. E. et al., A phase 1 study of the PI3Kδ inhibitor idelalisib in patients with relapsed/refractory mantle cell lymphoma (MCL). *Blood.* 2014; 123: 3398-405.

[57] Friedberg J. W., Sharman J., Sweetenham J., Johnston P. B., Vose J. M., et al., Inhibition of Syk with fostamatinib disodium has significant clinical activity in non-Hodgkin lymphoma and chronic lymphocytic leukemia. *Blood* 2012; 115: 2578-2585.

[58] Zhang J., Yang P. L., Gray N. S. Targeting cancer with small molecule kinase inhibitors. *Nat. Rev. Cancer.* 2009; 1:28-39.

[59] Friedberg J. W., Sharman J., Sweetenham J., Johnston P. B., Vose J. M. et al., Inhibition of Syk with fostamatinib disodium has significant

clinical activity in non-Hodgkin lymphoma and chronic lymphocytic leukemia. *Blood.* 2010; 115:2578-85.

[60] Efremov D. G., Laurenti L. The Syk kinase as a therapeutic target in leukemia and lymphoma. *Expert Opin Investig Drugs.* 2011; 20:623-36.

[61] Friedberg J. W., Sharman J., Sweetenham J., Johnston P. B., Vose J. M., et al., Inhibition of Syk with fostamatinib disodium has significant clinical activity in non-Hodgkin lymphoma and chronic lymphocytic leukemia. *Blood.* 2010; 115:2578-85.

[62] Benjamin D., Colombi M., Moroni C., Hall M. N. Rapamycin passes the torch: a new generation of mTOR inhibitors. *Nat. Rev. Drug Discovery* 2011; 10:868-880.

[63] Sehgal S. N., Baker H., Vezina C. Rapamycin (AY-22,989), a new antifungal antibiotic. II. Fermentation, isolation and characterization. *J. Antibiot.* 1975; 28:727-732.

[64] Vu C., Fruman D. A. Target of rapamycin signaling in leukemia and lymphoma. *Clin. Cancer Res.* 2010; 16:5374-5380.

[65] Witzig T. E., Geyer S. M., Ghobrial I., Inwards D. J., Fonseca R. et al., Phase II trial of single-agent temsirolimus (CCI-779) for relapsed mantle cell lymphoma. *J Clin Oncol.* 2005; 23:5347-5356.

[66] Hess G., Herbrecht R., Romaguera J., Verhoef G., Crump M. et al., Phase III study to evaluate temsirolimus compared with investigator's choice therapy for the treatment of relapsed or refractory mantle cell lymphoma. *J Clin Oncol.* 2009; 27:38220-3829.

[67] Goy A., Bernstein S. H., Kahl B. S., Djulbegovic B., Robertson M. J. et al., Bortezomib in patients with relapsed/refractory mantle cell lymphoma: updated time-toevent analysis of the multicenter phase 2 PINNACLE study. *Ann Oncol.* 2009; 20:520-252.

[68] Ruan J., Martin P., Furman R. R., Lee S. M., Cheung K. et al., Bortezomib plus CHOP-rituximab for previously untreated diffuse large B-cell lymphoma and mantle cell lymphoma. *J Clin Oncol.* 2011; 29:690-7.

[69] Dimopoulos M., Spencer A., Attal M., Prince H. M., Harousseau J. L. et al., Multiple Myeloma (010) Study Investigators Lenalidomide plus dexamethasone for relapsed or refractory multiple myeloma. *N. Engl. J. Med.* 2007; 357:2123-2132.

[70] List A., Dewald G., Bennett J., Giagounidis A, Raza A, et al., Myelodysplastic Syndrome-003 Study Investigators Lenalidomide in the myelodysplastic syndrome with chromosome 5q deletion. *N. Engl. J. Med.* 2006; 355:1456-1465.

[71] Martiniani R., Di Loreto V., Di Sano C., Lombardo A., Liberati A. M. Biological activity of lenalidomide and its underlying therapeutic effects in multiple myeloma. *Adv. Hematol.* 2012:842945.

[72] Zinzani P. L., Vose J. M., Czuczman M. S., Reeder C. B., Haioun C. et al., Phase II multicenter study of the safety and efficacy of single-agent lenalidomide in subjects with relapsed/refractory mantle cell lymphoma: long-term follow-up analysis of the NHL- 003 study. *Ann Oncol.* 2013; 24:2892-7.

[73] Goy A., Sinha R., Williams M. E., Kalayoglu Besisik S., Drach J. et al., Phase II multicenter study of singleagent lenalidomide in subjects with mantle cell lymphoma who relapsed or progressed after or were refractory to bortezomib: the MCL-001 "EMERGE" study. *J Clin Oncol.* 2013; 31:3688-95.

[74] Wang M., Fayad L., Wagner-Bartak N., Zhang L., Hagemeister F. et al., Lenalidomide in combination with rituximab for patients with relapsed or refractory mantle-cell lymphoma: a phase I/II clinical trial. *The Lancet Oncol.* 2012; 13:716-623.

[75] Demo S. D., Kirk C. J., Aujay M. A., Buchholz T. J., Dajee M. et al., Antitumor activity of PR-171, a novel irreversible inhibitor of the proteasome. *Cancer Res* 2007; 67:6383-91.

[76] Vij R., Kaufman J. L., Jakubowiak A. J., Stewart A. K., Jagannath S. et al., Carfilzomib: high single agent response rate with minimal neuropathy even in high-risk patients. *Blood* 2010; 116:1938.

[77] Vij R., Wang M., Kaufman J., L, Lonial S., Jakubowiak A. J. et al., An open-label, single-arm, phase 2 (PX-171-004) study of single-agent carfilzomib in bortezomib-naive patients with relapsed and/or refractory multiple myeloma. *Blood* 2012; 119:5661-70.

[78] Dasmahapatra G., Lembersky D., Son M. P., Attkisson E., Dent P. et al., Carfilzomib interacts synergistically with histone deacetylase inhibitors in mantle cell lymphoma cells *in vitro* and *in vivo*. *Mol Cancer Ther* 2011; 10: 1686-97.

[79] Hazar B., Paydas S., Zorludemir S., Sahin B., Tuncer I. Prognostic significance of microvessel density and vascular endothelial growth factor (VEGF) expression in non-Hodgkin's lymphoma. *Leuk Lymphoma.* 2003; 44:2089-93.

[80] Ruan J., Gregory S. A., Christos P., Martin P., Furman R. R., Coleman M., Leonard J. P. Long-term follow-up of R-CHOP with bevacizumab as initial therapy for mantle cell lymphoma: clinical and correlative results. *Clin Lymphoma Myeloma Leuk.* 2014; 14:107-13.

[81] Certo M., Del Gaizo Moore V., Nishino M., Wei G., Korsmeyer S. et al., Mitochondria primed by death signals determine cellular addiction to antiapoptotic BCL-2 family members. *Cancer Cell* 2006; 9:351-65.

[82] Ek S., Hogerkorp C. M., Dictor M., Ehinger M., Borrebaeck C. A. Mantle cell lymphomas express a distinct genetic signature affecting lymphocyte trafficking and growth regulation as compared with subpopulations of normal human B cells. *Cancer Res* 2002; 62:4398-405.

[83] Oltersdorf T., Elmore S. W., Shoemaker A. R., Armstrong R. C., Augeri D. J. et al., An inhibitor of Bcl-2 family proteins induces regression of solid tumours. *Nature* 2005; 435:677-81.

[84] Van Delft M. F., Wei A. H., Mason K. D., Vandenberg C. J., Chen L. et al., The BH3 mimetic ABT-737 targets selective Bcl-2 proteins and efficiently induces apoptosis via Bak/Bax if Mcl-1 is neutralized. *Cancer Cell* 2006; 10:389-99.

[85] Tahir S. K., Wass J., Joseph M. K., Devanarayan V., Hessler P. et al., Identification of expression signatures predictive of sensitivity to the Bcl-2 family member inhibitor ABT-263 in small cell lung carcinoma and leukemia/lymphoma cell lines. *Mol Cancer Ther* 2010; 9:545-57.

[86] Del Gaizo Moore V., Schlis K. D., Sallan S. E., Armstrong S. A., Letai A. BCL-2 dependence and ABT-737 sensitivity in acute lymphoblastic leukemia. *Blood* 2008; 111:2300-9.

In: Mantle Cell Lymphoma
Editor: Charles L. Schmidt
ISBN: 978-1-63482-363-0


*Chapter 4*

# Emerging Role of Novel Agents in the treatment of Mantle Cell Lymphoma

***Bridgette A. Kanz*[1]*, Mahsa S. Talbott*[1] *and Nishitha M. Reddy*[2*]**
Department of Pharmacology[1], Division of Hematology and Oncology[2],
Vanderbilt University Medical Center, Nashville, TN, US

## Abstract

The complex network of the malignant B cell with the tumor microenvironment and the constitutive activation of the B-cell receptor pathway promote survival and proliferation of malignant B cells. The downstream targets of the BCR pathway and the microenvironment are the other mediators of cell growth in B cell lymphoma. Recently, small molecule inhibitors that inhibit BCR associated pathways have shown encouraging activity in B cell lymphoma. The B cell receptor pathway therefore, has become an attractive prime target in several incurable lymphomas such as chronic lymphocytic leukemia and mantle cell

[*] Corresponding Author. Nishitha M. Reddy MD, 3927 The Vanderbilt Clinic, Vanderbilt-Ingram Cancer Center, Nashville, TN- 37232. Phone # (615) 936-0381; Fax # (615) 936-1812; Email: nishitha.reddy@vanderbilt.edu.

lymphoma. The growing body of knowledge on the efficacy of these agents and yet the lack of a comprehensive understanding of the potential targets and off target actions is intriguing.

In this chapter, we will review the safety, mechanism of action, efficacy and future directions of the targeted therapies in the management of mantle cell lymphoma.

**Keywords:** Mantle cell lymphoma; immunomodulatory drugs, specific kinase inhibitors

## Introduction

Mantle cell lymphoma (MCL) is a moderately aggressive B cell non-Hodgkin lymphoma (NHL) that accounts for 3-6% of all NHL. Historically, MCL has been associated with poor outcomes and high relapse rates, as it is incurable with conventional chemotherapy regimens [1]. Approximately 70% of patients present with stage IV disease at diagnosis [1]. The heterogeneity of this disease varies from a clinical presentation of being an indolent disease, to that of an aggressive lymphoma with multi organ involvement. [1, 2]

Younger, fit patients defined as patients 65 years of age or younger without significant comorbidities, are treated with dose intensified regimens [1, 2]. These include rituximab plus cyclophosphamide, doxorubicin, vincristine and prednisone (RCHOP), or hyperfractionated cyclophosphamide, doxorubicin, vincristine, and dexamethasone (R-HyperCVAD) with alternating rituximab and high-dose cytarabine and methotrexate (R- MA), followed by consolidative autologous stem cell transplant (ASCT). Response rates in these patients range from 40-65%.

Older patients or those with significant comorbidities are treated with less intense regimens. These regimens include bendamustine and rituximab (BR), fludarabine plus cyclophosphamide and rituximab (FCR), or R-CHOP alone. Response rates with these regimens vary from 73-92%. Patients who are not transplant candidates appear to derive a survival benefit with maintenance rituximab following chemotherapy [3]. The use of novel agents in combination with chemotherapy is under investigation. Bortezomib, a proteasome inhibitor, has been added to CHOP or hyper-CVAD with improved responses [4, 5].

Recent research has focused on treating relapsed and refractory MCL patients. Due to the rarity of the disease state, most data is based on small studies compared with historical controls [6, 7]. This chapter will review therapy specifically for relapsed or refractory patients, focusing on targeted therapies for the B-cell receptor (BCR) pathway.

The BCR pathway is integral in the survival and proliferation of malignant B cells. It is activated through antigen binding and is constitutively activated in MCL cell lines [8]. The BCR and its associated pathways relevant in MCL are now therapeutic targets of promising small molecule inhibitors. These targets include the mammalian target of rapamycin (mTOR), Bruton tyrosine kinase (BTK), phosphoinositide-3 kinase (PI3K), and cyclin-D molecule. Therapies explored in this chapter will include immunomodulators, mTOR inhibitors, BTK inhibitors, PI3K inhibitors, and cyclin-D inhibitors in terms of their mechanism of action, efficacy, postulated role and future directions.

# Immunomodulatory Agents in MCL

Thalidomide and lenalidomide are immunomodulating agents that have been investigated for the treatment of relapsed or refractory MCL. Their mechanism of action is not fully understood, but is thought to involve multiple aspects of the immune system such as tumor necrosis factor, integrins, T-cells, interleukins, production of immunological synapses and inhibition of angiogenesis [9].

## Clinical Activity of Immunomodulators in MCL

Thalidomide was evaluated in combination with rituximab for MCL with the rationale that the combination would target both the lymphoma as well as the immunologic microenvironment [10]. Sixteen patients with refractory or relapsed disease after CHOP or a CHOP-like regimen received rituximab 375 $mg/m^2$ once weekly for four weeks and thalidomide 200mg daily with a dose increase on day 15 to 400mg daily. Thalidomide was continued until disease progression. The overall response rate (ORR) was 81%. Peripheral neuropathy occurred in 44% of patients leading to discontinuation of therapy in one patient.

Results of the trial were limited by small patient numbers and potential side effects. In 2010, a study was published investigating the use of thalidomide with rituximab, prednisone, etoposide, procarbazine, and cyclophosphamide (RT-PEPC). RT-PEPC had shown an ORR of 73% in this study [11]. Phase II trials involving immunomodulators are detailed in Table 1.

Lenalidomide is a more potent immunomodulatory agent that thalidomide and therefore led to its investigation in various hematological malignancies. Rituximab, has successfully been used in multiple cancer regimens and has shown modest activity as monotherapy in patients with MCL [12, 13]. Preclinical studies combining rituximab and lenalidomide have shown to inhibit cell growth and induce apoptosis in MCL cell lines, with the combination exceeding the effect of either drug alone. Additional research showed a synergistic effect with this combination through lenalidomide increasing the antibody-dependent cellular toxicity of rituximab via activation of natural killer cells [14, 15].

Based on this preclinical data, multiple phase II trials were initiated. A combination phase 1/2 open label, single arm, clinical trial with relapsed or refractory MCL patients with CD20+ and cyclin D1 disease was conducted to determine the maximum tolerated dose (MTD) of lenalidomide and rituximab as well as its safety and efficacy [16]. Results showed the MTD of this regimen to be 20mg [16]. As such, the phase II trial conducted in 38 patients at this dose showed an ORR of 57%.

Two additional phase II studies were conducted utilizing lenalidomide in MCL patients. They are described in Table 2 (NHL 002 and NHL 003). These studies utilized a dosing regimen of 25mg of lenalidomide days 1-21 of a 28 day cycle. The ORR rates were 55% and 42% respectively [17, 19].

Long term follow up of MCL patients in NHL 003 was published after establishing more rigorous review of efficacy data. In this study, patients had a median of three prior treatments [19]. Central review of data review revealed an ORR of 35% (95% CI, 23-49%) with a 12% CR/CRu rate (95% CI, 5-24%). These results continued to support the initial data from NHL 003 and provided rationale for investigation of lenalidomide in MCL patients.

The EMERGE trial, or MCL 001, that led to its FDA approval in relapsed MCL, utilized the same regimen as NHL 002 and 003 and enrolled patients who had failed first line therapy for refractory or relapsed MCL and found an ORR of 28% (95% CI, 20-36%) [20].

Of note, ten patients (7%) reported venous thromboembolic events [20]. This calls into question whether prophylaxis is warranted. Upon further analysis, it was found that two events occurred in patients who did not receive anticoagulation and eight events occurred in patients who were anticoagulated, indicating further study is warranted to understand the necessity and optimizing anticoagulation with lenalidomide in this population.

Zaja and colleagues investigated its utility in combination with dexamethasone for MCL patients. Previously performed *in vitro* studies showed promising results with this combination and potential synergistic mechanisms of action resulting in decreased tumor proliferation, G0/G1 cell cycle arrest and increased apoptosis [21]. They enrolled patients with relapsed or refractory MCL in a multicenter, phase II study to receive lenalidomide 25mg on days 1-21 of each 28 day cycle and 40mg of dexamethasone on days 1, 8, 15, and 22 [22].

Results showed an overall response rate of 52%, or seventeen out of thirty-three patients, with a complete response seen in 18 of 33 patients. Authors concluded that their data supported the use of lenalidomide in MCL but postulated that using it in combination with dexamethasone may actually be detrimental as lenalidomide up-regulates the immune response while dexamethasone dampers it [22].

**Table 1. Clinical studies of immunomodulators in relapsed MCL**

| Author | Study | Included Patients | Therapy | ORR | ADR |
|---|---|---|---|---|---|
| Ruan et al. [11] | Phase II | 22 | RT-PEPC | 73% | Cytopenias, infections |
| Wang et al. [16] | Phase I | 14 | Rituximab + lenalidomide | NA | Cytopenias, thromboembolic events, fatigue, diarrhea, dyspnea, pain, pleural effusions |
| Wang et al. [16] | Phase II | 44 | Lenalidomide | 57% | |
| Wiernik et al. [17] | Phase II (NHL 002) | 15 | Lenalidomide | 53% | |
| Zinzani et al. [19] | Phase II (NHL 003) | 57 | Lenalidomide | 35% | |
| Goy et al. [20] | Phase II (MCL 001/ EMERGE) | 134 | Lenalidomide | 28% | |
| Zaja et al. [22] | Phase II | 33 | Lenalidomide + dexamethasone | 52% | Infections, febrile neutropenia |

RT-PEPC: Rituximab, thalidomide, prednisone, etoposide, procarbazine, and cyclophosphamide; ORR- Overall response rate; ADR: adverse drug reactions.

### Future Directions

Overall, results have shown that the combination of rituximab and lenalidomide is effective in MCL. The safety and efficacy profile reflects similarly to that of bortezomib, currently recommended first line for relapsed or refractory MCL [23, 24, 18]. Patients who were unable to tolerate bortezomib or who had failed bortezomib responded to lenalidomide and rituximab. This combination also compares favorably with lenalidomide as monotherapy as the combination improved the PFS of 5.7 months seen in NHL 003 to 8.8 months [16, 19]. Its activity as a single agent or in combination with rituximab led to its investigation in patients with previously untreated MCL, as initial induction and maintenance. In this chemotherapy-free treatment approach, 38 pts with advanced MCL were treated with 25 mg of lenalidomide. The ORR was 84%, with 52.6% achieving a CR. The estimated 2-yr PFS was 84%. This study demonstrates that future therapy may be geared towards a chemotherapy-free regimen in patients with MCL [25].

## The Role of BTK Inhibitors in MCL

Bruton tyrosine kinase (BTK) was named after Ogden Bruton who described a condition known as X-linked hypergammaglobulinemia (XLA) in the 1950s leading to lack of mature B cells and low serum immunoglobulin. This condition was due to a mutation in the Bruton tyrosine kinase blocking pre-B cell development and B-cell receptor signaling. The tyrosine kinase was named after Bruton in 1993 when the genetic cause of XLA was discovered [26]. Ibrutinib, formerly known as PCI-32765, mimics the action of XLA by taking advantage of BTK blockade to slow the proliferation and survival of B-cells. Interestingly, it does not reduce serum levels of immunoglobulin as XLA does [27]. This drug was recently approved in 2013 through accelerated Food and Drug Administration (FDA) approval for the treatment of relapsed or refractory MCL [28].

### Clinical Activity in MCL

Ibrutinib was initially developed as a treatment for rheumatoid arthritis and later led to the discovery of its anticancer activities in B-cell malignancies.

[26]. The phase I dosing trial established 2.5 mg/kg/day as the dose needed to engage BTK blockade but titration up to 12.5 mg/kg/day did not reach the MTD. Based on the side effects noted and the efficacy, 560mg daily was established as the dose moving forward in clinical trials. Nine of fifty patients enrolled in the phase I study had MCL, and seven of those nine saw ORR with three CRs [27]. Grade 3/4 toxicities were not common but included neutropenia (12.5%), thrombocytopenia (7.2%), and anemia (7.1%).

The international, open-label, phase II trial of ibrutinib enrolled patients with confirmed MCL and cyclin D1 overexpression and classic translocations. Patients had received one to five previous therapies and had progressed since their most recent regimen. The one hundred eleven enrolled patients were divided into two cohorts including patients who had received ≥ 2 cycles of bortezomib (n=48) and bortezomib naïve patients defined as < 2 cycles of bortezomib or none prior (n=63). Both cohorts received ibruitnib 560mg daily until progression of disease or intolerable adverse events [28].

Results illustrated an ORR of 68% with a median DOR of 17.5 months (95% CI, 15.8 months – not reached). Patients in both cohorts responded to therapy with CR of 19% in bortezomib naïve and 23% in bortezomib exposed [28]. Based on these results, ibrutinib was approved as first line therapy for relapsed or refractory MCL patients, adding a second option for prescribers besides bortezomib.

The medication was well tolerated with most adverse events being grade 1 or 2. Those that occurred at greater than 20% frequency included diarrhea, fatigue, nausea, peripheral edema, dyspnea, constipation, upper respiratory tract infection (URI), vomiting, and decreased appetite. Grade 3/4 hematologic events included neutropenia (16%), thrombocytopenia (11%), and anemia (10%). Four deaths were attributed to adverse events resulting from pneumonia, sepsis, and cardiac arrest. Treatment was stopped in eight patients (7%) due to adverse events [28].

During the initial phase of tumor reduction, a transient lymphocytosis was observed in the clinical studies. To dampen this response and improve the efficacy of ibrutinib, rituximab was added and evaluated in a phase II study of 50 patients. Rituximab was administered on days 1, 8, 15, 22 and then on day 1 of cycles 3-8, and thereafter once every other cycle for 2 years. Ibrutinib was dosed at 560 mg daily. In this phase II study, the ORR was 87% with 38% achieving a CR. Of note, in patients with a Ki-67 of <50%, the ORR was 100% [29].

Another BTK inhibitor, CC-292, is currently in phase I clinical trials. It is a covalent, irreversible BTK inhibitor but it also binds similar kinases with cysteine residues such as JAK3 and TEC. A dose finding trial established 2 mg/kg as a sufficient dose to inhibit BTK and is being investigated in the ongoing trial [30].

### Future Directions

Long term follow up of patients treated with BTK inhibitors is limited. Thus far, both primary and secondary resistance to ibrutinib has been described. Primary resistance occurs in about one-third of patients, with secondary resistance developing later in initial responders [31]. Research is now focused on understanding the mechanisms of resistance and ways to overcome this resistance. Recently, it has been noted that mutations in PIM1 kinase and ERBB4 kinases genes may be of interest in patients with primary resistance to ibrutinib therapy in MCL [32]. Future trials are focused on combining ibrutinib with other therapies that may inhibit or overcome this resistance.

Currently, ibrutinib is being investigated in various combinations including bendamustine and rituximab. Ibrutinib is also being studied as a single agent versus an mTOR inhibitor and in patients who have failed bortezomib [33].

## mTOR Inhibitors in MCL

The mammalian target of rapamycin (mTOR) is a serine threonine kinase that works to help control cell functions including proliferation, metabolism and survival by integrating signals from protein kinases and regulating further pathways downstream to enhance protein synthesis [34]. There are two complexes including mTORC1 and mTORC2. The first is the target of mTOR inhibitors including temsirolimus and everolimus [35].

In MCL, mTOR is constitutively activated by phosphoinositide kinases and AKT, described in further detail below. Because of its increased activation, mTOR in turn increases translation of cyclin D1, the hallmark feature of MCL [35].

## Clinical Activity in MCL

mTOR targets two main substrates including the eukaryotic initiation factor (eIF)4F complex and the ribosomal protein S6 kinases. Temsirolimus, an mTOR inhibitor approved in Europe for the treatment of relapsed or refractory MCL, works by binding the FK506-binding protein to form a complex that inhibits the active site of mTORC1 preventing the activation of these substrates [34].

It was approved based on one randomized controlled trial. Other trials involving mTOR inhibitors in MCL are summarized in Table 2 below [36]. Previous phase I and II trials had led to unclear optimal dosing so patients in this study were randomized to receive investigators choice of treatment, temsirolimus 175mg weekly for three doses followed by weekly doses of 25mg or weekly doses of 75mg. The ORRs were 2%, 6% and 22% respectively with median PFS of 1.9, 3.4 and 4.8 months [37].

From this study, several conclusions were drawn. First, temsirolimus is superior to standard treatments in relapsed and refractory patients but is still only modestly effective as monotherapy. Next, the dosing schedule of 175mg/75mg was superior to 175mg/25mg. Finally, thrombocytopenia was confirmed as the major toxicity of temsirolimus, as it had also emerged in previous trials. This side effect is to be expected in patients who have most likely received previous intensive regimens. Other side effects included asthenia, anemia and diarrhea [37, 36].

**Table 2. Clinical studies of mTOR inhibitors in MCL**

<table>
<tr><th>Author</th><th>Study</th><th>Patients</th><th>Therapy</th><th>ORR</th><th>ADR</th></tr>
<tr><td>Witzig et al. [38]</td><td>Phase II</td><td>35</td><td>Temsirolimus</td><td>38%</td><td rowspan="2">Cytopenias, hyperglycemia, mucositis, fatigue</td></tr>
<tr><td>Ansell et al. [39]</td><td>Phase II</td><td>27</td><td>Temsirolimus</td><td>41%</td></tr>
<tr><td>Renner et al. [40]</td><td>Phase II</td><td>35</td><td>Everolimus</td><td>20%</td><td rowspan="3">Thrombocytopenia, neutropenia, anemia</td></tr>
<tr><td>Witzig et al. [41]</td><td>Phase II</td><td>77</td><td>Everolimus</td><td>32%</td></tr>
<tr><td>Wang et al. [42]</td><td>Phase II</td><td>58</td><td>Everolimus</td><td>8.6%</td></tr>
</table>

The specificity of the mTOR inhibitors for the mTORC1 complex limits their use. As mTOR is activated by AKT, mTORC1 acts on AKT as negative feedback [34]. There are various forms of resistance that circumvent this pathway that increase the activity of AKT to perpetuate cellular proliferation. Hypotheses of these resistance mechanisms include upregulation of AKT through gene amplification and direct activation of AKT through mTORC2. Because of these issues, there are dual inhibitors being developed.

### Future Directions

The mTOR kinase is only one part of a larger pathway. Through various efforts, researchers have found that inhibiting a part of this pathway is not sufficient to stop the progression of MCL [43].

Further therapy with mTOR inhibitors is limited by drug resistance pathways and microenvironment signals. For this reason, Rosich et al., studied the efficacy of NVP-BEZ235, which inhibits kinase activity of PI3K, mTORC1 and mTORC2. In MCL cell lines, this drug was more effective than a PI3K inhibitor plus mTORC1 inhibitor. This indicates that therapy targeting multiple kinases involved in this pathway will be an important aspect of the future of MCL therapy [43].

## MCL and PI3K Inhibitors

There are three classes of phosphoinositide-3 kinases, each with their own functionality. Class IA has the most relevance in oncology and is comprised of a p85 regulatory subunit as well as a p110 catalytic subunit [44]. Both subunits have isoforms including α, β, and δ p110 and α, β, γ and δ p85, each providing a potential therapeutic target. PI3K activation comes from an upstream signal, usually mediated by a receptor tyrosine kinase.

In MCL, PI3K mediated phosphorylation activates a threonine/serine kinase, AKT, as well as the mTOR, as noted above. The activation of these pathways helps stabilize the production of cyclin D1 and pathogenesis of MCL [45, 46, 47, 48]. Specifically, the PI3K δ isoform has shown to be more active in BCR signaling and promotion of B-cell function and proliferation.

## Activity of PI3K in MCL

Idelalisib, or GS-1101, is a small molecule inhibitor of the PI3K p110δ isoform. In preclinical research, it has been shown to block PI3K/AKT signaling and promote apoptosis [49, 50]. The phase I 48-week dose-escalation study evaluated dosing schemas from 50mg-350mg daily or twice daily in various B-cell malignancies including acute myeloid leukemia, multiple myeloma and MCL. Forty patients with MCL were enrolled with a median of four prior treatments, including rituximab (100%), alkylating agents (98%), anthracyclines (88%), and bortezomib (60%) [51].

In terms of safety, the MTD was not reached and adverse events were not correlated with the dose [51]. Most adverse events were grades 1 and 2. Overall, the most common adverse events included diarrhea (40%), nausea (32.5%), pyrexia (27.5%), fatigue (25%), rash (22.5%), decreased appetite (20%), and URI (20%). The most common adverse events greater than grade 3 included diarrhea (17.5%), decreased appetite (15%), and pneumonia (10%). Adverse events resulted in discontinuation in 18% of patients. Elevations in liver enzymes were observed in 60% of patients (24/40) with 20% occurring at a grade 3 or above severity level. As such, dose adjustments are recommended at grade 3.

A unique effect seen with idelalisib is mobilization of cells from the bone marrow resulting in transient lymphocytosis. In the MCL subset of patients, only five patients (12.5%) had an increase in lymphocyte count greater than three-fold their baseline, with normalization achieved over two to three months [51].

In this study, the ORR among MCL patients was 40% (95% CI, 24.9-56.7%). Higher doses (≥150mg twice daily) were associated with a higher response rate and the 2 patients that achieved a CR were both receiving 300mg of idelalisib daily [51]. Unfortunately, the duration of response was only 2.7 months (95% CI, 1-8.1 months). Median PFS was associated with number of prior treatments; For patients with < 6 prior treatments, the median PFS was 8.2 months (range 0.9-20.1 months) versus patients with ≥ 6 regimens who had a median PFS of 3.7 months (range 0.03-14.8 months).

## Future Directions

The authors of this study postulated that resistance to, or progression of, disease after PI3Kδ inhibitors may be due to overexpression of other PI3K isoforms, particularly PI3K p110α [43]. Dual inhibitor therapy may produce more durable responses in future studies. Regardless, idelalisib showed positive results in this phase I study and warrants phase II investigation in this population. The MTD was not identified but future studies will utilize 150mg twice daily due to plateau efficacy rates above this dose and considerations of adverse event profiles [51]. Idelalisib was approved in 2014 for the treatment of patients with chronic lymphocytic leukemia with rituximab, relapsed follicular B-cell NHL, and relapsed small lymphocytic lymphoma but does not carry an indication for MCL.

Several other molecules are being investigated for use in the PI3K pathway. Pan-isoform inhibitor buparlisib, or BKM120, is the furthest along in phase II and III studies [52]. Buparlisib binds to the ATP binding site in PI3K in both a competitive and non-competitive manner [44]. In a phase I study, the most common side effects seen were gastrointestinal, rash, fatigue and hyperglycemia [53]. Hyperglycemia has been seen in other pan PI3K inhibitors as well due to PI3K's role in insulin signaling [52]. Of note, this drug caused mood disturbances at both the MTD and lower doses and should be used with caution in patients with a history of depression [44]. Buparlisib is currently being investigated for use in HER2- breast cancer patients but may potentially play a role in other B-cell malignancies.

Overall, the PI3K pathway presents an enticing target for B-cell malignancies. However, the various molecules developed thus far have shown lukewarm results leaving investors wondering if they are worth the investment to further develop [52]. Other therapeutic options in this pathway include novel dual mechanistic drugs targeting multiple steps in the B-cell receptor pathway, such as PI3K and mTOR, to help reduce drug resistance [44]. One such drug currently under investigation is NVP-BEZ235.

NVP-BEZ235 is an imidazoquinoline derivative that inhibits both the PI3K as well as mTOR pathways, including mTORC1 and mTORC2 [54]. It has shown benefit in multiple lymphoid malignancies including acute leukemia and MCL [55]. In a comparison against BKM120 and everolimus (an mTOR inhibitor), NVP-BEZ235 was superior at reducing phosphorylation of AKT and inducing apoptosis in MCL cell lines [43]. NVP-BEZ235 also showed efficacy in the microenvironment modulating angiogenesis and cytokine signaling. This indicates that targeting multiple levels of the PI3K pathway may help reduce resistance and maintain remission in MCL patients. Further research is needed in this area to confirm these hypotheses.

# Cyclin-D1 Inhibitors in MCL

The cyclin D proteins include three proteins, cyclin D1, D2, and D3 that help regulate cell cycle. They form complexes with kinases and phosphorylate retinoblastoma protein, which in turn regulates the E2F proteins that control the start of the cell cycle. Cyclin D is mainly active in the G1 to S phase transition of the cell cycle [56]. Cyclin D1 is overexpressed in MCL and has been shown to be necessary to cell function along with cyclin D3. Because of this, it is postulated that therapies targeting both cyclins would be most effective.

## Clinical Activity of Cyclin Inhibitors in MCL

Cyclin D1 expression and actions are not well understood and have been difficult to target. Multiple drugs developed thus far may play a role in modulating cyclin D1 but the exact mechanisms of action are not understood. Bortezomib downregulates the level of cyclin D1 proteins but does not affect the RNA production [57]. Finally, histone deacetylase inhibitors, such as vorinostat, have been effective at reducing cyclin D1 protein levels thought to be mediated through PI3K inhibition.

The other opportunity to modify this pathway includes targeting the associated kinases that complex with cyclin D proteins. One such therapy, flavopiridol or alvocidib, inhibits cyclin D kinase 1 (CDK1) and was studied in a phase I trial with fludarabine and rituximab. This study included ten patients with MCL who achieved a median PFS of 21.9 months and 80% ORR. However, utilization of this therapy is limited by severe myelosuppression, with 68% of the study population enduring grade 3 or 4 leukopenia and 66% experiencing grade 3 or 4 neutropenia [58].

## Future Directions

A follow up study in patients with chronic lymphocytic leukemia is investigating the use of flavopiridol via a pharmacokinetic directed dosing schedule to assess if some side effects can be reduced. Another cyclin inhibitor, curcumin, is currently being investigated in combination with bortezomib [57]. Curcumin is an herbal plant flavonoid that has shown down regulation of both cyclin D1 and D3 at the level of transcription in both multiple myeloma and MCL lines [59].

# Conclusion

The landscape of therapy for relapsed and refractory MCL is rapidly changing. Despite recent progress, prognosis remains poor and it remains a disease with several challenges to overcome. First, MCL is a disease that despite an initial response to therapy, residual cells remain in the marrow or gastrointestinal tract, making MCL prone to recurrence. Improved methods to detect minimal residual disease (MRD) at these sites and overcoming MRD with novel agents either by continuing therapy or by deepening initial response are considerable strategies. Second, it is characteristic for drug resistance to emerge as a cause for relapsed MCL. This may be related to the interaction of the tumor infiltrating cells in the microenvironment. Stromal cells found in bone marrow and secondary lymphoid sites promote the proliferation and possibly drug resistance from cross-talk between microenvironment and the lymphoma cells. The mechanism by which this occurs is not well understood. Third, the heterogeneity in the biology of this disease, with the blastoid variant of MCL, presenting as a highly proliferative disease that almost universally carries a poor prognosis, is a challenge when considering treatment. Future studies using DNA technology and next-generation sequencing may play a role in our understanding of this complex environment. With advancements in effective new therapies, future research may focus on utilizing novel therapies earlier in care especially considering their toxicity profiles and incidence of MCL in the elderly population. As our understanding of these drugs advances, drug sequence and duration of novel therapy would support continued investigation in MCL.

# References

[1] Rajguru, S. and Kahl, B. (2014), "Emerging Therapy for the Treatment of Mantle Cell Lymphoma", *Journal of the National Comprehensive Cancer Network*, Vol. 12, pp. 111–118.

[2] Shah, B. and Martin, P. (2012), "Mantle Cell Lymphoma: A Clinically Heterogenous Disease in Need of Tailored Approaches", *Cancer Control*, Vol. 19 No. 3, pp. 227-235.

[3] Kluin-Nelemans HC, Hoster E, Hermine O, et al. Treatment of older patients with mantle-cell lymphoma. The New England journal of medicine 2012;367:520-31.

[4] Till, B. et al. (2014), "Phase II Trial of R-CHOP Plus Bortezomib Induction Therapy Followed by Bortezomib Maintenance for Previously Untreated Mantle Cell Lymphoma: SWOG 0601", *56$^{th}$ ASH Annual Meeting and Exposition,* Abstract # 149.

[5] Chang, J. (2014), "Phase 2 study of VcR-CVAD with maintenance rituximab for untreated mantle cell lymphoma: an Eastern Cooperative Oncology Group Study (E1405)", *Blood,* Vol. 123 No. 11, pp. 1665-73.

[6] Vose, J.M. (2013), "Mantle Cell Lymphoma: 2013 Update on Diagnosis, Risk-Stratification and Clinical Managment", *American Journal of Hematology*, Vol. 88, pp. 1083–1088.

[7] DeVita, Vincent, Lawrence, Theodore and Rosenberg, Steven. (2009), *DeVita, Hellman, and Rosenberg's Cancer: Principles & Practice of Oncology*, Lippincott Williams & Wilkins, Baltimore, MD, 2nd Edition.

[8] Galan-Perez, P. (2011), "Mantle Cell Lymphoma: biology, pathogenesis and the molecular basis of treatment in the genomic era", *Blood*, Vol. 117 No. 1, pp. 26–38.

[9] Skarbnik, A. (2013), "Therapies for Mantle Cell Lymphoma: Current Challenges and a Brighter Future", *Discovery Medicine*, Vol. 18 No. 82.

[10] Kaufmann, H. and Raderer, M. (2004), "Antitumor activity of rituximab plus thalidomide in patients with relapsed/refractory mantle cell lymphoma", *Blood*, Vol. 104, pp. 2269–2271.

[11] Ruan, J. and Martin, P. (2010), "Durable Responses With the Metronomic Rituximab and Thalidomide Plus Prednisone, Etoposide, Procarbazine, and Cyclophosphamide Regimen in Elderly Patients With Recurrnet Mantle Cell Lymphoma", *Cancer*, Vol. 116, pp. 2655–2664.

[12] Ghielmini, M. (2005), "Effect of single-agent rituximab given at the standard schedule or as prolonged treatment in patients with mantle cell lymphoma: a study of the Swiss Group for Clinical Cancer Research (SAKK)", *J Clin Oncol*, Vol. 23, pp. 705–711.

[13] Foran, J. (2000), "European phase II study of rituximab (chimeric anti-CD20 monoclonal antibody) for patients with newly diagnosed mantle-cell lymphoma and previously treated mantle-cell lymphoma,

immunocytoma, and small B-cell lymphocytic lymphoma", *J Clin Oncol*, Vol. 18, pp. 17–324.

[14] Bartlett, J. (2007), "Lenalidomide and pomalidomide strongly enhance tumor cell killing in vitro during antibody-dependent cellular cytotoxicity (ADCC) mediated by trastuzumab, cetuximab and rituximab.", *Proc Am Soc Clin Oncol*, Vol. 25, p. 3023.

[15] Wu, L. (2008), "Lenalidomide enhances natural killer cell and monocyte-mediated antibody-dependent cellular cytotoxicity of rituximab-treated CD20+ tumor cells", *Clin Cancer Res*, Vol. 14, pp. 4650–4657.

[16] Wang, M. and Fayad, L. (2012), "Lenalidomide in combination with rituximab for patients with relapsed or refractory mantle-cell lymphoma: a phase 1/2 clinical trial", *Lancet Oncology*, Vol. 13, pp. 716–723.

[17] Wiernik, P. and Lossos, I. (2008), "Lenalidomide Monotherapy in Relapsed or Refractory Aggressive Non-Hodgkin's Lymphoma", *Journal of Clinical Oncology*, Vol. 26 No. 30, pp. 4952–4957.

[18] Witzig, T.E. and Vose, J.M. (2011), "An international phase II trial of single-agent lenalidomide for relapsed or refractory aggressive B-cell non-Hodgkin's lymphoma", *Annals of Oncology*, Vol. 22, pp. 1622–1627.

[19] Zinzani, P.L. and Vose, J.M. (2013), "Long-term follow-up of lenalidomide in relapsed/refractory mantle cell lymphoma: subset analysis of the NHL-003 study", *Annals of Oncology*, Vol. 24, pp. 2892–2897.

[20] Goy, A. and Sinha, R. (2013), "Single-agent Lenalidomide in Patients With Mantle-Cell Lymphoma Who Relapsed or Progressed After or Were Refractory to Bortezomib: Phase II MCL-001 (EMERGE) Study", *Journal of Clinical Oncology*, Vol. 1 No. 29, pp. 3688–3695.

[21] Z, Q. (2011), "Lenalidomide synergizes with dexamethasone to induce growth arrest and apoptosis of mantle cell lymphoma cells in vitro and in vivo", *Leuk Res*, Vol. 35 No. 3, pp. 380–386.

[22] Zaja, F. and De Luca, S. (2012), "Salvage treatment with lenalidomide and dexamethasone in relapsed/refractory mantle cell lymphoma: clinical results and effects on microenvironment and neo-angiogenic biomarkers", *Haematologica*, Vol. 97 No. 3, pp. 416–422.

[23] Fisher, R. (2006), "Multicenter phase II study of bortezomib in patients with relapsed or refractory mantle cell lymphoma", *J Clin Oncol*, Vol. 24, pp. 4867–74.

[24] Goy, A. (2009), "Bortezomib in patients with relapsed or refractory mantle cell lymphoma: updated time-to-event analysis of the multicenter phase 2 PINNACLE study", *Ann Oncol*, Vol. 20, pp. 520–25.

[25] Ruan, J. et al. (2014), "Sustained Remission with the Combination Biologic Doublet of Lenalidomide Plus Rituximab as Initial Treatment for Mantle Cell Lymphoma: A Multi-Center Phase II Study Report", *56th ASH Annual Meeting and Exposition,* Abstract # 625.

[26] Ponader, S. and Burger, J. (2014), "Bruton's Tyrosine Kinase: From X-Linked Agammaglobulinemia Toward Targeted Therapy for B-Cell Malignancies", *Journal of Clinical Oncology*, Vol. 32, pp. 1830–39.

[27] Advani, R. and Buggy, J. (2012), "Bruton Tyrosine Kinase Inhibitor Ibrutinib (PCI-32765) Has Significant Activity in Patients with Relapsed/Refractory B-Cell Malignancies", *Journal of Clinical Oncology*, Vol. 1, pp. 88–94.

[28] Mahajan, S. (1999), "Rational design and synthesis of a novel antileukemic agent targeting Bruton's tyrosine kinase (BTK), LFM-A13 [alpha-cyano-beta-hydroxy-beta-methyl-N-(2,5-dibromophenyl) propenamide]", *J Biol Chem*, Vol. 274, pp. 9587–9599.

[29] Wang, M. et al. (2014), "Ibrutinib and Rituximab Are an Efficacious and Safe Combination in Mantle cell Lymphoma: Preliminary Results from a Phase II Clinical Trial", *56th ASH Annual Meeting and Exposition,* Abstract # 627.

[30] Evans, E. (2013), "Inhibition of Btk with CC-292 provides early pharmacodynamic assessment of activity in mice and humans", *J Pharmacol Exp Ther*, Vol. 346, pp. 219–228.

[31] Ma, J. and Lu, P. (2014), "Characterization of ibrutinib-sensitive and -resistant mantle lymphoma cells", *British Journal of Haematology*, Vol. 166, pp. 849–861.

[32] Balasubramanian, S. et al. (2014), "Mutational Analysis of Patients with Primary Resistance to Single-Agent Ibrutinib in Relapsed or Refractory Mantle Cell Lymphoma (MCL)", *56th ASH Annual Meeting and Exposition,* Abstract # 78.

[33] Chen, Y., Wang, M. and Romaguera, J. (2014), "Current regimens and novel agents for mantle cell lymphoma", *British Journal of Hematology*, Vol. 167, pp. 3–18.

[34] Samad, N., Younes, A. (2010) "Temsirolimus in the treatment of relapsed or refractory mantle cell lymphoma", *OncoTargets and Therapy*, Vol. 3, pp. 167-178.

[35] Hess, G. (2009), "Temsirolimus for the treatment of mantle cell lymphoma", *Expert Rev Hematol*, Vol. 2 No. 6, pp. 61-640.
[36] Dreyling, M., Geisler, C., et al. (2014) "Newly diagnosed and relapsed mantle cell lymphoma: ESMO Clinical Practice Guidelines for diagnosis, treatment and follow-up", *Ann Oncol*, Vol. 25 Supplement 3, pp. iii83-iii92.
[37] Hess, G., Herbrecht, R. and Romaguera, J. (2009), "Phase III Study to Evaluate Temsirolimus compared with investigator's choice therapy for the treatment of relapsed or refractory mantle cell lymphoma," *J Clin Oncol*, Vol. 27 No. 23, pp. 3822-3829.
[38] Witzig, T., Geyer, S., Ghobrieal, I. (2005), "Phase II trial of single-agent temsirolimus (CCI-779) for relapsed mantle cell lymphoma," *J Clin Oncol,* Vol. 23 No. 23, pp. 532-5356.
[39] Ansell, S., Inwards, D., Rowland, K. (2008), "Low-dose single-agent temsirolimus for relapsed mantle cell lymphoma: a Phase 2 trial in the North Central Cancer Treatment Group," *Cancer*, Vol. 113 No. 3, pp. 508-514.
[40] Renner, C., Zinzani, P. et al. (2012), "A multicenter phase II trial (SAKK36/06) of single-agent everolimus (RAD001) in patients with relapsed or refractory mantle cell lymphoma," *Haematologica*, Vol. 97, pp. 1085-1091.
[41] Witzig, T., Reeder, C., et al. (2011), "A phase II trial of the oral mTOR inhibitor everolimus in relapsed aggressive lymphoma," *Leukemia*, Vol. 25, pp. 341-32.
[42] Wang, M., Popplewell, L., et al. (2014), "Everolimus for patients with mantle cell lymphoma refractory to or intolerant of bortezomib: multicenter, single-arm, phase 2 study," *Br J Haematol,* Vol. 165, pp. 510-518.
[43] Rosich, L. and Montraveta, A. (2014), "Dual PI3K/mTOR inhibition is required to effectively impair microenvironment survival signals in mantle cell lymphoma", *Oncotarget*, Vol. 5 No. 16, pp. 6788–6800.
[44] Kurtz, J.-E. and Ray-Coquard, I. (2012), "PI3 Kinase Inhibitors in the Clinic: An Update", *Anticancer Research*, Vol. 32, pp. 2463–220.
[45] Rizzatti, E. (2005), "Gene expression profiling of mantle cell lymphoma cells reveals aberrant expression of genes from the PI3K-AKT, WNT and TGFbeta signalling pathways", *Br J Haematol*, Vol. 130 No. 4, pp. 5116–526.

[46] Dal Col, J. (2008a), "Distinct functional significance of Akt and mTOR constitutive activation in mantle cell lymphoma.", *Blood*, Vol. 111 No. 10, pp. 5142–5151.

[47] Dal Col, J. (2008b), "GSK-3beta inhibition: at the crossroad between Akt and mTOR constitutive activation to enhance cyclin D1 protein stability in mantle cell lymphoma," *Cell Cycle*, Vol. 7 No. 18, pp. 2813–2816.

[48] Prasad, A. (2009), "Styryl sulfonyl compounds inhibit translation of cyclin D1 in mantle cell lymphoma cells", *Oncogene*, Vol. 28 No. 12, pp. 1518–1528.

[49] Lannutti, B. (2011), "CAL-101, a p110delta selective phosphatidylinositol-3-kinase inhibitor for the treatment of B-cell malignancies, inhibits PI3K signaling and cellular viability", *Blood*, Vol. 117 No. 2, pp. 591–594.

[50] Herman, S. (2011), "The role of phosphatidylinositol 3-kinase-delta in the immunomodulatory effects of lenalidomide in chronic lymphocytic leukemia.", *Blood*, Vol. 117 No. 16, pp. 4323–4327.

[51] Kahl, B. and Spurgeon, S. (2014), "A phase 1 study of the PI3K delta inhibitor idelalisib in patients with relapsed/refractory mantle cell lymphoma (MCL)", *Blood*, Vol. 123, pp. 3398–3405.

[52] Cho, D. (2013), "Despite Lukewarm Clinical Benefit of PI3K Inhibitors, Optimism Remains Regarding Biomarkers and Combination Therapy", American Society of Clinical Oncology.

[53] Rodon, J. and Brana, I. (2014), "Phase I dose-escalation and -expansion study of buparlisib (BKM120), an oral pan-Class I PI3K inhibitor, in patients with advanced solid tumors", *Investigational New Drugs*, Vol. 32, pp. 670–681.

[54] Maira, S. (2008), "Identification and characterization of NVP-BEZ235, a new orally available dual phosphatidylinositol 3-kinase/mammalian target of rapamycin inhibitor with potent in vivo antitumor activity", *Mol Cancer Ther*, Vol. 7, pp. 1851–1863.

[55] Muller, A. (2013), "Concurrent inhibition of PI3K and mTORC1/ mTORC2 overcomes resistance to rapamycin induced apoptosis by down-regulation of Mcl-1 in mantle cell lymphoma", *Int J Cancer*, Vol. 133, pp. 1813–1824.

[56] Hasanali, Z. and Sharma, K. (2012), "Flipping the cyclin D1 switch in mantle cell lymphoma", *Best Practice and Research Clinical Haematology*, Vol. 25, pp. 143–152.

[57] Klier, M. (2011), "Crosstalk between cyclins D1 and D3 in mantle cell level at the transcriptional and postranscriptional levels", *ASH Annu Meet Abstr*, Vol. 118, p. 1373.
[58] Lin, T. (2009), "Flavopiridol, Fludarabine, and Rituximab in Mantle Cell Lymphoma and Indolent B-Cell Lymphoproliferative Disorders", *Journal of Clinical Oncology*, Vol. 28, pp. 418–423.
[59] Singh, A. (2011), "Curcumin nanodisk-induced apoptosis in mantle cell lymphoma", *Leuk Lymphoma*, Vol. 52, pp. 1537–43.

In: Mantle Cell Lymphoma
Editor: Charles L. Schmidt
ISBN: 978-1-63482-363-0


*Chapter 5*

# Current Place of Proteasome Inhibitors in the Treatment of Mantle Cell Lymphoma

***Panagiotis J. Vlachostergios**[1] *and Rajeev L. Balmiki*[2]**
[1]Department of Internal Medicine,
Lutheran Medical Center, Brooklyn, NY, US
[2]Department of Hematology/Oncology,
Lutheran Medical Center, Brooklyn, NY, US

## Abstract

Mantle cell lymphoma (MCL) is an uncommon non-Hodgkin (NHL) lymphoma subtype with distinct features in terms of its clinical presentation and prognosis which are usually characterized by diffuse extranodal disease, including spleen and bone marrow involvement as well as an intermediate to high MCL international prognostic score. Elucidation of MCL underlying molecular aberrations not only resulted in the emergence of a key role for cyclin D1 and intracellular protein turnover regulation but has also introduced a rational of targeted therapeutic approaches, of which proteasome inhibitors have become an

* Correspondence: Panagiotis J. Vlachostergios M.D., Ph.D.; Department of Internal Medicine; Lutheran Medical Center; 150 55th Street, Brooklyn; NY 11220, New York, USA; E-mail: pvlachostergios@lmcmc.com.

essential part. Bortezomib is the first proteasome inhibitor which was established as part of FDA-approved therapy for relapsed/refractory MCL in 2006. Since then much progress has been noted with accumulating preclinical and early clinical evidence suggesting additive or/and synergistic activity of bortezomib and newer proteasome inhibitors with cytotoxic and targeted agents, including but not limited to rituximab, histone deacetylase inhibitors, mTOR inhibitors and cyclin-dependent kinase inhibitors. A growing number of combination studies is currently under progress in MCL patients with the aim of better understanding and framing the use of proteasome inhibitors in the continuum of treatment approaches for the management of MCL.

**Keywords:** Mantle cell ymphoma, proteasome inhibitors, bortezomib, cyclin D1, targeted therapy

# Introduction

Mantle cell lymphoma (MCL) is a distinct subtype of non-Hodgkin lymphoma (NHL), accounting for 3% to 6% of all NHLs, with a median age at diagnosis of 68 years and a significant male predominance. Most patients present at advanced stage and with a high-intermediate or high International Prognostic Index (IPI) score. Diffuse lymphadenopathy, splenomegaly, and bone marrow involvement are usually present at diagnosis, as well as extranodal disease in the majority of patients, particularly with gastrointestinal involvement [1].

Overexpression of cyclin D1 is the central molecular aberration of the disease, leading to cell cycle dysregulation [1]. The cyclin D1 gene is located at 11q13, and its product drives cell cycle progression from G1 to S phase. Aberrant expression of cyclin D1 occurs either through the (11;14)(q13;q32) translocation which juxtaposes the DNA coding sequence for cyclin D1 at 11q13 with the immunoglobulin heavy-chain joining region at 14q32 [2, 3] or via mutations and/or genomic deletions that affect the 3' untranslated region of cyclin D1 resulting in the expression of truncated mRNA [4]. These truncations stabilize the cyclin D1 RNA transcript, resulting in increased cyclin D1 mRNA and increased protein levels [5, 6].

The MCL IPI (MIPI) score is an important clinical tool for prognostication and classifies patients into different categories using 4 independent factors (age, performance status, lactate dehydrogenase, and WBC count), based on which patients are divided into low-risk (44% of patients), intermediate risk (35% of patients with a median OS of 51 months), and high-risk (21% of patients with a median OS of 29 months). The cell proliferative index (Ki-67) is another prognostic indicator [1], while increased truncated relative to full-length cyclin D1 mRNA is also associated with poor clinical outcomes [4-6].

## The Molecular Basis of Proteasome Inhibition in MCL

Cyclin D1, cell-cycle control, and DNA damage pathways are considered central in molecular pathogenenesis and evolution of MCL. In addition, several other signaling pathways promoting proliferation, evasion of apoptosis and downregulation of immune surveillance have been suggested to contribute to the MCL phenotype, including the B-cell receptor (BCR), PI3K/AKT/mammalian target of rapamycin (mTOR), nuclear factor-kappa B (NF-κB), tumor necrosis factor (TNF), Hedgehog, and WNT, and BCL-2 family apoptotic pathways [7].

The ubiquitin-proteasome system (UPS) consists the main non-lysosomal pathway through which intracellular proteins are degraded, and has 3 types of proteolytic activity: chymotrypsin-like, trypsin-like, and caspase-like, each localized to a distinct 20S proteasome subunit. Bortezomib is the first peptide boronic acid, acting as a reversible inhibitor primarily of the chymotrypsin-like activity, that was approved for treatment of patients with relapsed or refractory MCL [8].

The mechanism of anticancer action of bortezomib on MCL cells has been extensively investigated, with primary hypotheses supporting a central role of inhibition of NF-κB signaling [9]. However, newer studies suggest the mechanism underlying bortezomib-induced apoptosis in MCL is up-regulation of the BH3-only protein NOXA. The accumulation of undegraded, polyubiquitinated proteins induces an endoplasmic reticulum stress and generation of reactive oxygen species, triggering a cellular stress response the transcriptional component of which prominently involves the activation of the transcription factor NRF2. The latter was found to be significantly stronger in bortezomib-sensitive tumors than in tumors of patients with inferior responses. Ultimately, NOXA is induced by a combination of decreased ubiquitination of histone H2A that facilitates access to the NOXA gene (PMAIP1) promoter, and of joint binding of transcription factors ATF3 and ATF4 that drive its transcription. Ultimately, NOXA triggers BAK- and BAX-dependent mitochondrial apoptosis [10].

An additional mechanism of action for bortezomib's anti-cancer activity has been proposed in non-MCL (breast) cancer cells and involves the amplification of the proapoptotic function of cyclin D1 acting as a repressor of the STAT3/Bcl-XL survival axis, thus raising the possibility that cyclin D1 levels may be a marker for predicting responses [11].

## Bortezomib in Newly Diagnosed MCL

The combination of bortezomib with standard chemoimmunotherapy was tested in a phase I/II study. 36 patients with previously untreated MCL received R-CHOP with addition of escalating doses of bortezomib (0.7, 1.0, or 1.3 mg/m$^2$). The overall response rate (ORR) was 81% in the intent-to-treat population, with a 64% complete response (CR)/unconfirmed CR (CRu) rate. The 2-year progression-free survival (PFS) rate was 44% (95% CI, 27%–60%) and the 2-year overall survival (OS) rate was 86% (95% CI, 70%–94%). These results suggest an improvement in the CR/CRu rate when bortezomib is combined with R-CHOP [12].

Bortezomib was also tested in the modified R-hyperCVAD regimen (VcR-CVAD) in a phase II study (ECOG E1405). 75 patients with previously untreated MCL received VcR-CVAD for 6 cycles. The ORR was 95% (95% CI, 87%–99%), with a CR rate of 68% (95% CI 57%–79%). The 3-year PFS and OS rates were 72% and 88%, respectively. No grade 3/4 peripheral neuropathy was observed as a lower dosage schedule of bortezomib and vincristine (1.3 mg/m$^2$ and 1.0 mg, respectively) was used [13].

In a preliminary report of a randomized trial of VcR-CAP versus R-CHOP in 482 transplant-ineligible patients with previously untreated MCL, VcR-CAP resulted in superior median PFS (25 versus 14 months; hazard ratio 0.63, 95% CI 0.50-0.79) [14, 15]. Rates of overall and complete response were 88 and 44 percent, respectively. VcR-CAP was associated with higher rate of severe (grade ≥4) neutropenia (70 versus 52 percent) and thrombocytopenia (32 versus 1 percent), and a higher incidence of herpes zoster reactivation (4.6 versus 0.8 percent). The greater toxicity with this regimen limits its use in older patients not eligible for transplant.

Collectively, for upfront therapy of MCL, bortezomib is an acceptable alternative in combination with chemoimmunotherapy (VcR-CAP) to conventional chemoimmunotherapy regimens (BR, R-CHOP, R-CVP).

## Bortezomib in Relapsed/Refractory MCL

There have been several prospective phase II trials of bortezomib in patients with relapsed or refractory (R/R) MCL demonstrating ORR from 29 to 50 percent and CR rates from 4 to 8 percent [16-21]. The median duration of response is approximately 10 months.

The multicenter phase II PINNACLE study was the landmark study to establish the role of bortezomib in R/R MCL, leading to FDA approval in 2006. The 155 patients of the study were treated with bortezomib at 1.3 $mg/m^2$ intravenously on days 1, 4, 8, and 11 of a 21-day cycle, with 141 patients assessable for response. The median number of prior therapies was 1. The ORR was 33% (8% CR/CRu) and the median duration of response was 9.2 months. Grade 3 or higher peripheral neuropathy was seen in 13% of patients [19].

Another phase II prospective trial evaluated bortezomib in 29 patients with MCL, 13 of whom had received no prior therapy. The ORR was 46% with a median response duration of 10 months. Response rates were similar in previously untreated and recurrent disease [20].

A prospective trial of bortezomib that included 24 patients with R/R lymphoma reported responses in 7, including one complete response [18]. Another phase II trial of bortezomib in 40 patients reported similar ORR (50 versus 43 percent) and PFS (5.6 versus 3.9 months) for patients with R/R disease, respectively [8].

In another phase II trial, the combination of bortezomib with gemcitabine was found to be effective in patients with rR/R MCL with an ORR of 60% and a median PFS of 11.4 months [22].

A recent phase II clinical trial tested the addition of bortezomib to the bendamustine-rituximab (BR) regimen showing encouraging PFS results and leading to the initiation of randomized trials comparing the BR-bortezomib combination with BR alone [23].

Collectively, bortezomib is a standard of care for the treatment of patients with R/R MCL who have received at least one prior therapy.

# Other Bortezomib – Containing Combinations in MCL

The combination of bortezomib with the immunomodulatory agent lenalidomide was both active and tolerated in a phase II study of patients with R/R MCL [24].

Bortezomib was also combined with radioimmunotherapy, namely ibritumomab tiuxetan in a phase I study that reported responses in 80% of patients with MCL [25].

Bortezomib was shown to enhance fludarabine activity by inhibiting DNA repair and induction apoptosis in Bcl-2– overexpressing cells. When combined in a phase I study, a PR was reported in one patient with MCL, but cytopenias resulting in treatment discontinuation occurred in two other MCL patients [26].

In a phase I study that included heavily pretreated patients with MCL bortezomib was combined with cytarabine, and dexamethasone, resulting in an ORR was 50%, but at the cost of grade 3–4 hematologic toxicities [27].

Bortezomib, rituximab, fludarabine, and liposomal doxorubicin were combined in R/R MCL patients, producing an ORR of 73% [28].

Bortezomib, rituximab, and hyperfractionated cyclophosphamide was another combination tested in a phase I study in elderly patients (72–84 years of age) reporting a 75% ORR [29].

A phase II study of bortezomib, rituximab, and dexamethasone (BORID) in 16 heavily pretreated MCL patients reported a 69% RR [30], while addition of doxorubicin and chlorambucil to BORID resulted in an 80% RR [31].

Addition of bortezomib to hyper-CVAD with high-dose rituximab or rituximab, methotrexate, and cytarabine (R-M/A) resulted in objective responses in 15 patients without additional toxicities compared to the ones that would be expected without bortezomib [32].

## Dosing Schedule of Bortezomib

The recommended dose of bortezomib for R/R MCL is administration every 3 weeks, with an i.v. bolus of bortezomib administered over 3–5 seconds on days 1, 4, 8, and 11. A s.c. formulation of bortezomib was recently approved with the same dosing guidelines as the i.v. formulation. After the first eight doses, extended therapy can be administered in 5-week cycles on days 1, 8, 15, and 22. Randomized comparisons did not show significant difference in efficacy between the twice-weekly schedule and the once-weekly schedule [30, 33-37]. However, weekly dosing of bortezomib in combination regimens seems to be better tolerated [33, 38-40].

## Toxicity of Bortezomib

The adverse events reported for bortezomib use in MCL are similar to those previously reported in patients with multiple myeloma and most commonly include anorexia, nausea and vomiting, peripheral neuropathy, cutaneous reactions, neutropenia, and thrombocytopenia.

Combination of bortezomib with rituximab in patients with R/R MCL has demonstrated high rates of toxicity. A phase I/II trial of bortezomib plus rituximab in 42 patients with R/R MCL, follicular lymphoma, or Waldenström macroglobulinemia resulted in discontinuation of treatment in 16 of 42 patients [33]. In another study, among 14 MCL patients treated with bortezomib plus rituximab, 52% developed grade 3 neurologic toxicity [22]. Bortezomib plus rituximab and pulsed dexamethasone in 16 patients with R/R MCL resulted in severe (grade 3/4) toxicities including thrombocytopenia (38%), fatigue (19%), and peripheral neuropathy (13%), despite a high RR of 81% (44 % complete) with a median OS of 39 months [23].

In a gene expression analysis of the HOVON-65/GMMG-HD4 trial on newly diagnosed multiple myeloma, upregulation of genes RHOBTB2 (involved in drug-induced apoptosis), CPT1C (mitochondrial dysfunction), and SOX8 (peripheral nervous system development) in the myeloma samples was associated with early-onset bortezomib-induced neuropathy, whereas upregulation of SOD2 and MYO5A (involved in nervous system development) was associated with late onset bortezomib-induced neuropathy [38]. Likewise, genetic analysis of peripheral blood from the same patients revealed that significant single-nucleotide polymorphisms in the genes caspase 9, ALOX12, and IGF1R were associated with early-onset neuropathy, whereas MBL2, PPARD, ERCC3, and ERCC4 were associated with late-onset neuropathy. These interesting findings need to be validated in patients with MCL and in prospective or randomized trials, as they may be useful in individualizing bortezomib treatment. Finally, a comparison of s.c. and i.v. administration of bortezomib in a phase III trial of relapsed multiple myeloma demonstrated less peripheral neuropathy of the s.c. arm (38% vs. 53% for any neuropathy, and 6% vs. 16% for grade III/IV neuropathy), with no difference in ORR, PFS, or OS [39, 40].

## Newer Proteasome Inhibitors in MCL

Newer proteasome inhibitors are in development, including the irreversible inhibitors carfilzomib and marizomib (salinosporamide A, NPI-0052) and the oral inhibitors ONX-0912 and MLN-9708, however none is approved for treatment of MCL [41-44]. Carfilzomib has been approved for the treatment of patients with multiple myeloma who have received at least 2 prior therapies, including bortezomib and an immunomodulatory agent (e.g., thalidomide or lenalidomide) [45].

Carfilzomib has a similar mechanism of action with bortezomib but it binds proteasomes irreversibly and is selective for the chymotrypsin-like active site [46]. Marizomib also binds the proteasome irreversibly [47], leading to activation of caspase-8 [48, 49] and potentiation of apoptosis [50], but it inhibits all three sites for up to 7 days and it may be a more potent inhibitor of NF-κB than bortezomib [51, 52]. However, it remains to be determined whether or not differences in binding kinetics influence clinical efficacy and safety [53]. ONX-0912 (previously PR-047) has a chemical structure similar to that of carfilzomib and is also selective for the chymotrypsin-like active site [54] and is orally available. MLN-9708 is a boron-containing proteasome inhibitor which is also orally available, with better tissue distribution than bortezomib [44].

Data from a phase I trial reports that responses to marizomib were found in patients with bortezomib-refractory multiple myeloma [55].

Ixazomib (MLN-9708) is the first oral proteasome inhibitor to enter clinical investigation in myeloma patients. Results from a phase I trial with ixazomib monotherapy suggest durable disease control and good tolerance and rare peripheral neuropathy in heavily pretreated R/R myeloma patients [56].

Delanzomib (CEP-18770) is another oral boronate-based reversible proteasome inhibitor on phase I/II clinical testing. Delanzomib has shown in vitro proteasome-inhibitory activity similar to that of bortezomib in hematologic and solid tumor cell lines and primary cells from myeloma patients [57]. Finally, orally administered oprozomib (ONX-0912) has equivalent antitumor activity to intravenously administered carfilzomib in human tumor xenograft and mouse syngeneic models and its po administration twice daily is currently being investigated in early clinical trials [58, 59].

## Proteasome Inhibitors in Combination with Novel Targeted Therapies in MCL

Preclinical assessments of combinations of bortezomib and histone deacetylase inhibitors (HDACi) have identified several potential mechanisms resulting in synergistic antitumor activity with NF-κB playing a central role. Thus, bortezomib through blocking IκBα degradation and inhibiting activation of NF-κB and NF-κB target genes, it enhances HDACi-mediated reactive oxygen species and apoptosis in MCL cell lines [60].

Carfilzomib/HDACi regimens were found to be active against bortezomib-resistant MCL cells. The combination of carfilzomib and vorinostat resulted in a pronounced reduction in tumor growth compared with single agent treatment in an MCL xenograft model associated with enhanced apoptosis [61].

The combination of bortezomib and cyclin-dependent kinase (CDK)-inhibitor alvocidib decreased myeloid cell leukemia 1 protein (Mcl-1) expression, and increased proapoptotic Bak in MCL cell lines [62]. The combination of bortezomib and alvocidib is tolerable and appears to be efficacious in patients with R/R multiple myeloma or indolent non-Hodgkin lymphoma, including MCL [63].

Bortezomib is also being evaluated in combination with the orally bioavailable mTOR inhibitor everolimus, in a phase I study of patients with R/R MCL and other indolent lymphomas (NCT0067112) [64].

In preclinical studies with bortezomib, the farnesyltransfersase inhibitors tipifarnib, and lonafarnib demonstrated additive and/or synergistic activity in MCL models [65-67].

The pan-bcl-2 inhibitor obatoclax and bortezomib had synergistic antitumor activity against MCL cell lines, through decreasing bortezomib-induced Mcl-1 and enhancing Noxa-mediated displacement of Bak from Mcl-1 [68, 69]. Bortezomib is being investigated with obatoclax in phase I–II studies in patients with R/R MCL (NCT00407303). Data from the MCL trial indicated that the combination is active and has acceptable toxicity profile [70]. Objective responses occurred in 4/13 (31%) evaluable patients (three complete and one partial response). Six patients (46%) had stable disease lasting ≥ 8 weeks. Thus, obatoclax and bortezomib combination is feasible, but the synergy demonstrated in preclinical models was not confirmed [71].

# Conclusion

Single-agent bortezomib is approved for use for MCL and has been shown to have activity for other forms of NHL as well. Early clinical studies of other proteasome inhibitors such as carfilzomib and marizomib have not yet provided compelling support for their use as single agents, but more mature data are needed before their single-agent safety and activity can be determined. The mechanisms of action of proteasome inhibitors are distinct from those of other treatments, and preclinical evidence suggests that they can be additive or synergistic with many standard treatments for MCL, including targeted agents, with an acceptable safety profile [67]. This is particularly significant, considering the elevated average age of patients affected by MCL, and the efforts being made in order to find a less toxic but still effective first and second line treatment tailored according to patient and disease molecular characteristics [68].

# References

[1] Rajguru S, Kahl BS. Emerging therapy for the treatment of mantle cell lymphoma. *J Natl Compr Canc Netw* 2014;12:1311-8.

[2] Harris NL, Jaffe ES, Stein H, et al. A revised European-American classification of lymphoid neoplasms: a proposal from the International Lymphoma Study Group. *Blood* 1994; 84:1361.

[3] Raffeld M, Jaffe ES. bcl-1, t(11;14), and mantle cell-derived lymphomas. *Blood* 1991; 78:259.

[4] Wiestner A, Tehrani M, Chiorazzi M, et al. Point mutations and genomic deletions in CCND1 create stable truncated cyclin D1 mRNAs that are associated with increased proliferation rate and shorter survival. *Blood* 2007; 109:4599.

[5] Chen RW, Bemis LT, Amato CM, et al. Truncation in CCND1 mRNA alters miR-16-1 regulation in mantle cell lymphoma. *Blood* 2008; 112:822.

[6] Shakir R, Ngo N, Naresh KN. Correlation of cyclin D1 transcript levels, transcript type and protein expression with proliferation and histology among mantle cell lymphoma. *J Clin Pathol* 2008; 61:920.

[7] Pérez-Galán P, Dreyling M, Wiestner A. Mantle cell lymphoma: biology, pathogenesis, and the molecular basis of treatment in the genomic era. *Blood* 2011;117:26-38.

[8] O'Connor OA, Moskowitz C, Portlock C, et al. Patients with chemotherapy-refractory mantle cell lymphoma experience high response rates and identical progression-free survivals compared with patients with relapsed disease following treatment with single agent bortezomib: results of a multicentre Phase 2 clinical trial. *Br J Haematol* 2009;145:34-9.

[9] Yang DT, Young KH, Kahl BS, Markovina S, Miyamoto S. Prevalence of bortezomib-resistant constitutive NF-kappaB activity in mantle cell lymphoma. *Mol Cancer* 2008;7:40.

[10] Pérez-Galán P, Roué G, Villamor N, Montserrat E, Campo E, Colomer D. The proteasome inhibitor bortezomib induces apoptosis in mantle-cell lymphoma through generation of ROS and Noxa activation independent of p53 status. *Blood* 2006;107:257-64.

[11] Ishii Y, Pirkmaier A, Alvarez JV, et al. Cyclin D1 overexpression and response to bortezomib treatment in a breast cancer model. *J Natl Cancer Inst* 2006;98:1238-47.

[12] Ruan J, Martin P, Furman RR, et al. BortezBZmib plus CHOP-rituximab for previously untreated diffuse large B-cell lymphoma and mantle cell lymphoma. *J Clin Oncol* 2011;29:690–697.

[13] Chang JE, Li H, Smith MR, et al. Phase 2 study of VcR-CVAD with maintenance rituximab for untreated mantle cell lymphoma: an Eastern Cooperative Oncology Group study (E1405). *Blood* 2014;123:1665–1673.

[14] http://www.accessdata.fda.gov/drugsatfda_docs/label/2014/021602s040lbl.pdf (Accessed on October 13, 2014).

[15] Cavilli F, Rooney B, Pei L, et al. Randomized phase 3 study of rituximab, cyclophosphamide, doxorubicin, and prednisone plus vincristine (R-CHOP) or bortezomib (VR-CAP) in newly diagnosed mantle cell lymphoma (MCL) patients (pts) ineligible for bone marrow transplantation (BMT). *J Clin Oncol* 2014; 32:5s.

[16] Goy A, Younes A, McLaughlin P, et al. Phase II study of proteasome inhibitor bortezomib in relapsed or refractory B-cell non-Hodgkin's lymphoma. *J Clin Oncol* 2005; 23:667.

[17] O'Connor OA, Wright J, Moskowitz C, et al. Phase II clinical experience with the novel proteasome inhibitor bortezomib in patients with indolent non-Hodgkin's lymphoma and mantle cell lymphoma. *J Clin Oncol* 2005; 23:676.

[18] Strauss SJ, Maharaj L, Hoare S, et al. Bortezomib therapy in patients with relapsed or refractory lymphoma: potential correlation of in vitro sensitivity and tumor necrosis factor alpha response with clinical activity. *J Clin Oncol* 2006; 24:2105.

[19] Fisher RI, Bernstein SH, Kahl BS, et al. Multicenter phase II study of bortezomib in patients with relapsed or refractory mantle cell lymphoma. *J Clin Oncol* 2006; 24:4867.

[20] Belch A, Kouroukis CT, Crump M, et al. A phase II study of bortezomib in mantle cell lymphoma: the National Cancer Institute of Canada Clinical Trials Group trial IND.150. *Ann Oncol* 2007; 18:116.

[21] Gerecitano J, Portlock C, Moskowitz C, et al. Phase 2 study of weekly bortezomib in mantle cell and follicular lymphoma. *Br J Haematol* 2009; 146:652.

[22] Baiocchi RA, Alinari L, Lustberg ME, et al. Phase 2 trial of rituximab and bortezomib in patients with relapsed or refractory mantle cell and follicular lymphoma. *Cancer* 2010.

[23] Lamm W, Kaufmann H, Raderer M, et al. Bortezomib combined with rituximab and dexamethasone is an active regimen for patients with relapsed and chemotherapy-refractory mantle cell lymphoma. *Haematologica* 2011; 96:1008.

[24] Morrison VA, Johnson JL, Jung S et al. A phase II trial of bortezomib plus lenalidomide for relapsed/refractory mantle cell lymphoma (MCL) (CALGB 50501): Results of a planned interim analysis. *J Clin Oncol* 2010;28(15 suppl):Abstract 8106.

[25] Beaven AW, Shea TC, Moore DT et al. A phase I study evaluating ibritumomab tiuxetan (Zevalin) in combination with bortezomib (Velcade) in relapsed/refractory mantle cell and low grade B-cell non-Hodgkin lymphoma. *Leuk Lymphoma.* 2012;53:254 –258.

[26] Snell M, Koc ON, Bahlis NJ et al. A phase I trial of PS-341 and fludarabine for relapsed and refractory indolent non-Hodgkin's lymphoma and chronic lymphocytic leukemia. *J Clin Oncol* 2006;24(18 suppl):Abstract 7580.

[27] Weigert O, Weidmann E, Mueck R et al. A novel regimen combining high dose cytarabine and bortezomib has activity in multiply relapsed

and refractory mantle cell lymphoma—long-term results of a multicenter observation study. *Leuk Lymphoma* 2009;50:716–722.
[28] Orciuolo E, Buda G, Pelosini M et al. Fludarabine, bortezomib, Myocet and rituximab chemotherapy in relapsed and refractory mantle cell lymphoma. *Br J Haematol* 2010;148:810–812.
[29] Musto PM, Guariglia R, Pietrantuono G et al. A pilot study with rituximab, bortezomib and hyper-fractionated cyclophosphamide (RBC regimen) for the treatment of advanced mantle cell lymphoma in elderly patients. *Haematologica* 2008;93(suppl 1):Abstract 0273.
[30] Gerecitano J, Portlock CS, Hamlin PA Jr et al. Rituximab, cyclophosphamide, bortezomib and prednisone (R-CBorP): Final results of a phase I trial evaluating two dosing schedules and the safety of overlapping pegfilgrastim in patients with relapsed/refractory indolent and mantle cell lymphomas [abstract]. *Blood* 2009;114:Abstract 3708.
[31] Friedberg JW, Vose JM, Kelly JL et al. The combination of bendamustine, bortezomib, and rituximab for patients with relapsed/refractory indolent and mantle cell non-Hodgkin lymphoma. *Blood* 2011;117:2807–2812.
[32] Drach J, Kaufmann H, Pichelmayer O et al. Bortezomib, rituximab, and dexamethasone (BORID) as salvage treatment in relapsed/refractory mantle cell lymphoma: Sustained disease control in patients achieving a complete remission [abstract]. *Blood* 2007;110:Abstract 2578.
[33] Agathocleous A, Rohatiner A, Rule S et al. Weekly versus twice weekly bortezomib given in conjunction with rituximab, in patients with recurrent follicular lymphoma, mantle cell lymphoma and Waldenström macroglobulinaemia. *Br J Haematol* 2010;151:346 –353.
[34] Ribrag V, Tilly H, Casasnovas O et al. Final results of a randomized phase 2 multicenter study of two bortezomib schedules in patients with recurrent or refractory follicular lymphoma. Groupe d'Etude des Lymphomes de l'Adulte (GELA) study FL-05 [abstract]. *Blood* 2010;116:Abstract 768.
[35] de Vos S, Goy A, Dakhil SR et al. Multicenter randomized phase II study of weekly or twice-weekly bortezomib plus rituximab in patients with relapsed or refractory follicular or marginal-zone B-cell lymphoma. *J Clin Oncol* 2009;27:5023–5030
[36] Agathocleous A, Rule S, Johnson P et al. Preliminary results of a phase I/II study of weekly or twice weekly bortezomib in combination with rituximab, in patients with follicular lymphoma, mantle cell lymphoma

and Waldenstrom's macroglobulinaemia [abstract]. *Blood* 2007;110:Abstract 2559.
[37] Moosmann PR, Heizmann M, Kotrubczik N et al. Weekly treatment with a combination of bendamustine and bortezomib in relapsed or refractory indolent non-Hodgkin's lymphoma: A single-center phase 1/2 study [abstract]. *Blood* 2008;112:Abstract 1574.
[38] Broyl A, Corthals SL, Jongen JL, et al. Mechanisms of peripheral neuropathy associated with bortezomib and vincristine in patients with newly diagnosed multiple myeloma: a prospective analysis of data from the HOVON-65/GMMG-HD4 trial. *Lancet Oncol* 2010;11:1057–65.
[39] Moreau P, Pylypenko H, Grosicki S, et al. Subcutaneous versus intravenous administration of bortezomib in patients with relapsedmultiplemyeloma: a randomised, phase 3, non-inferiority study. *Lancet Oncol* 2011;12:431–40.
[40] Deng C, Lee S, O'Connor OA. New strategies in the treatment of mantle cell lymphoma. *Clin Cancer Res.* 2012;18:3499-508.
[41] O'Connor OA, Stewart AK, Vallone M et al. A phase 1 dose escalation study of the safety and pharmacokinetics of the novel proteasome inhibitor carfilzomib (PR-171) in patients with hematologic malignancies. *Clin Cancer Res* 2009;15:7085–7091.
[42] Ruiz S, Krupnik Y, Keating M et al. The proteasome inhibitor NPI-0052 is a more effective inducer of apoptosis than bortezomib in lymphocytes from patients with chronic lymphocytic leukemia. *Mol Cancer Ther* 2006;5:1836 –1843.
[43] Roccaro AM, Sacco A, Aujay M et al. Selective inhibition of chymotrypsin-like activity of the immunoproteasome and constitutive proteasome in Waldenstrom macroglobulinemia. *Blood* 2010;115:4051–4060.
[44] Kupperman E, Lee EC, Cao Y et al. Evaluation of the proteasome inhibitor MLN9708 in preclinical models of human cancer. *Cancer Res* 2010;70:1970 –1980.
[45] http://www.aetna.com/cpb/medical/data/800_899/0845.html.
[46] Kuhn DJ, Chen Q, Voorhees PM et al. Potent activity of carfilzomib, a novel, irreversible inhibitor of the ubiquitin-proteasome pathway, against preclinical models of multiple myeloma. *Blood* 2007;110:3281–3290.
[47] Williamson MJ, Blank JL, Bruzzese FJ et al. Comparison of biochemical and biological effects of ML858 (salinosporamide A) and bortezomib. *Mol Cancer Ther 2006*;5:3052–3061.

[48] Chauhan D, Catley L, Li G et al. A novel orally active proteasome inhibitor induces apoptosis in multiple myeloma cells with mechanisms distinct from bortezomib. *Cancer Cell* 2005;8:407– 419.
[49] Miller CP, Ban K, Dujka ME et al. NPI-0052, a novel proteasome inhibitor, induces caspase-8 and ROS dependent apoptosis alone and in combination with HDAC inhibitors in leukemia cells. *Blood* 2007;110:267–277.
[50] Ahn KS, Sethi G, Chao TH et al. Salinosporamide A (NPI-0052) potentiates apoptosis, suppresses osteoclastogenesis, and inhibits invasion through downmodulation of NF-B regulated gene products. *Blood* 2007;110:2286 –2295.
[51] Chauhan D, Hideshima T, Anderson KC. A novel proteasome inhibitor NPI-0052 as an anticancer therapy. *Br J Cancer* 2006;95:961–965.
[52] Potts BC, Albitar MX, Anderson KC et al. Marizomib, a proteasome inhibitor for all seasons: Preclinical profile and a framework for clinical trials. *Curr Cancer Drug Targets* 2011;11:254 –284.
[53] Dick LR, Fleming PE. Building on bortezomib: Second-generation proteasome inhibitors as anti-cancer therapy. *Drug Discov Today* 2010;15:243–249.
[54] Chauhan D, Singh AV, Aujay M et al. A novel orally active proteasome inhibitor ONX 0912 triggers in vitro and in vivo cytotoxicity in multiple myeloma. *Blood* 2010;116:4906–4915.
[55] Richardson PG, Spencer A, Cannel P, et al. Phase 1 Clinical Evaluation of Twice-Weekly Marizomib (NPI-0052), a Novel Proteasome Inhibitor, in Patients with Relapsed/Refractory Multiple Myeloma (MM). *Blood.* 2011; 118:140–141.
[56] Richardson PG, Baz R, Wang LH, et al. Investigational Agent MLN9708, An Oral Proteasome Inhibitor, in Patients (Pts) with Relapsed and/or Refractory Multiple Myeloma (MM): Results From the Expansion Cohorts of a Phase 1 Dose-Escalation Study. *Blood.* 2011; 118:140.
[57] Molineaux SM. Molecular Pathways: Targeting Proteasomal Protein degradation in Cancer. *Clinical Cancer Research.* 2012; 18:15–20.
[58] Chauhan D, Singh AV, Aujay M, et al. A novel orally active proteasome inhibitor ONX 0912 triggers in vitro and in vivo cytotoxicity in multiple myeloma. *Blood.* 2010; 116:4906–4915.
[59] Buac D, Shen M, Schmitt S, et al. From bortezomib to other inhibitors of the proteasome and beyond. *Curr Pharm Des.* 2013;19:4025-4038.

[60] Heider U, Kaiser M, Zavrski I, et al. Synergistic interaction of the histone deacetylase inhibitor SAHA with the proteasome inhibitor bortezomib in mantle cell lymphoma [abstract]. *Blood* 2006;108:710–1a.

[61] Dasmahapatra G, Lembersky D, Son MP, et al. Carfilzomib interacts synergistically with histone deacetylase inhibitors in mantle cell lymphoma cells in vitro and in vivo. *Mol Cancer Ther.* 2011;10:1686-1697.

[62] Kapanen A, Tucker C, Chikh G, Bally M, Klasa R. Cell based assays completed with the mantle cell lymphoma cell lines Z138 and NCEB-1 indicate that combinations of bortezomid and flavopiridol interact to achieve synergistic activity [abstract]. *Blood* 2005;106:678a.

[63] Holkova B, Kmieciak M, Perkins EB, et al. Phase I trial of bortezomib (PS-341; NSC 681239) and "nonhybrid" (bolus) infusion schedule of alvocidib (flavopiridol; NSC 649890) in patients with recurrent or refractory indolent B-cell neoplasms. *Clin Cancer Res.* 2014;20:5652-5662.

[64] Wright JJ. Combination therapy of bortezomib with novel targeted agents: an emerging treatment strategy. *Clin Cancer Res.* 2010;16:4094-4104.

[65] Yanamandra N, Colaco NM, Parquet NA, et al. Tipifarnib and bortezomib are synergistic and overcome cell adhesion-mediated drug resistance in multiple myeloma and acute myeloid leukemia. *Clin Cancer Res* 2006;12:591–599.

[66] Kaufman JL, David E, Torre C, Sinha R, Lonial S. Enhanced levels of apoptosis by combination of farnesyl transferase inhibition (tipifarnib) and proteasome inhibition (bortezomib) in myeloma cell lines and primary myeloma cells and its mechanistic effects on Akt and caspase pathways [abstract]. *Blood* 2005;106:451a.

[67] Rolland D, Camara-Clayette V, Barbarat A, et al. Farnesyltransferase inhibitor R115777 inhibits cell growth and induces apoptosis in mantle cell lymphoma. *Cancer Chemother Pharmacol* 2008;61:855–863.

[68] Perez-Galan P, Roue G, Villamor N, et al. The BH3-mimetic GX15–070 synergizes with Bortezomib in Mantle Cell Lymphoma by enhancing Noxa-mediated activation of Bak. *Blood* 2007;109:4441–9.

[69] Perez-Galan P, Roue G, Lopez-Guerra M, et al. BCL-2 phosphorylation modulates sensitivity to the BH3 mimetic GX15–070 (Obatoclax) and reduces its synergistic interaction with bortezomib in chronic lymphocytic leukemia cells. *Leukemi*a 2008;22:1712–1720.

[70] Goy A, Ford P, Feldman T, et al. A phase 1 trial of the pan bcl-2 family inhibitor obatoclax mesylate (GX15–070) in combination with bortezomib in patients with relapsed/refractory mantle cell lymphoma [abstract]. *Blood* 2007;110:2569.
[71] Goy A, Hernandez-Ilzaliturri FJ, Kahl B, Ford P, Protomastro E, Berger M. A phase I/II study of the pan Bcl-2 inhibitor obatoclax mesylate plus bortezomib for relapsed or refractory mantle cell lymphoma. *Leuk Lymphoma.* 2014 Dec;55:2761-2768.

# Index

## C



## D

## E



## F



## G



## H

## I



## J



## K

## L



## M



## N

## O



## P



## R

## S



## T

## U



## V



## W



## Y